SHORT CASES *for the* MRCPCH

PASS PAEDIATRICS

Commissioning Editor: Ellen Green
Project Development Manager: Hannah Kenner
Project Manager: Frances Affleck
Design Direction: George Ajayi

SHORT CASES *for the* MRCPCH

PASS PAEDIATRICS

Angela Thomson
BSc MBChB MRCP(Edin) MRCPCH MD

Specialist Registrar in Paediatric Oncology, University College London Hospital, London, UK

Hamish Wallace
MD FRCPCH FRCP(Edin)

Consultant Paediatric Oncologist, Royal Hospital for Sick Children, Edinburgh, UK

Terence Stephenson
BSc BM BCh DM FRCP(London) FRCPCH

Professor of Child Health and Dean of the Faculty of Medicine and Health Sciences, University Hospital, Nottingham, UK

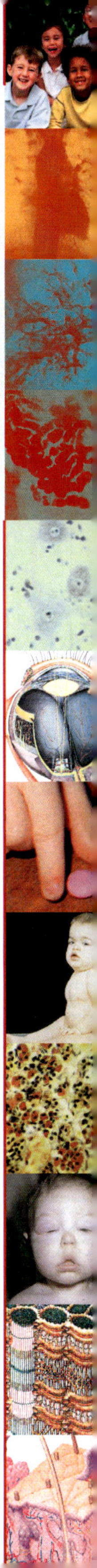

ELSEVIER
CHURCHILL LIVINGSTONE

EDINBURGH LONDON NEW YORK PHILADELPHIA ST LOUIS SYDNEY TORONTO 2005

ELSEVIER
CHURCHILL
LIVINGSTONE
An imprint of Elsevier Limited

First published 2005

ISBN 0 443 07040 7

British Library Cataloguing in Publication Data
A catalogue record for this book is available from the British Library

Library of Congress Cataloging in Publication Data
A catalog record for this book is available from the Library of Congress

Notice
Medical knowledge is constantly changing. Standard safety precautions must be followed, but as new research and clinical experience broaden our knowledge, changes in treatment and drug therapy may become necessary or appropriate. Readers are advised to check the most current product information provided by the manufacturer of each drug to be administered to verify the recommended dose, the method and duration of administration, and contraindications. It is the responsibility of the practitioner, relying on experience and knowledge of the patient, to determine dosages and the best treatment for each individual patient. Neither the Publisher nor the authors assume any liability for any injury and/or damage to persons or property arising from this publication.

The Publisher

The publisher's policy is to use **paper manufactured from sustainable forests**

Printed and bound by CPI Group (UK) Ltd, Croydon, CR0 4YY
Transferred to Digital Print 2011

Preface

This book has been inspired by our experience in teaching doctors for post-graduate paediatric examinations and our own experience in passing them. While this book is not a textbook it is specifically designed to aid learning and revision for the clinical parts of the new (2004) MRCPCH exam and the DCH exam.

The recognition and assessment of clinical signs is at the heart of all post-graduate paediatric examinations. The purpose of this book is to introduce you to common clinical scenarios that you might be faced with in examinations and give you the opportunity to improve your ability to explain and interpret your findings.

There is however no substitute for supervised clinical practise under the guidance of an experienced clinician. We hope you will enjoy our book and that it will become a friend and constant companion on your journey into higher training in paediatrics.

AT
HW
TS

Acknowledgements

We are grateful to parents and children for the use of the clinical photographs shown throughout this book, and to the authors of the texts from which some images have been taken for their kind permission to reproduce these figures.

Contents

1 INTRODUCTION

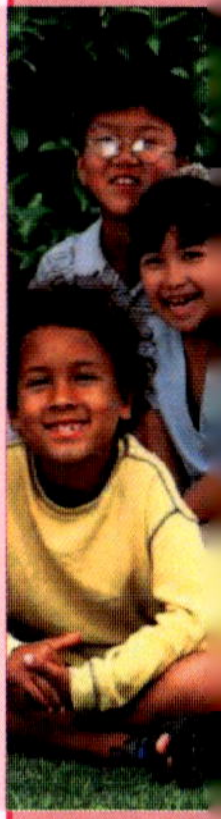

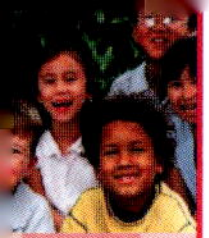

Acquiring the MRCPCH is one of the requirements for entry to higher specialist training in paediatrics in the UK. The format for the MRCPCH examination is continuously reviewed. However, irrespective of the details of how the examination is conducted, the clinical skills required to undertake a 'short case' (or the equivalent of a 'short case' at one of the stations of an OSCE) will remain essential for all aspiring paediatricians. Up to date information about the MRCPCH can be obtained from:

Royal College of Paediatrics and Child Health
50 Hallam Street
London W1W 6DE
Tel: 020 7307 5600
Fax: 020 7307 5601
Website: www.rcpch.ac.uk/exams

THE NEW MRCPCH CLINICAL EXAMINATION CIRCUIT

From October 2004, the separate examination of a long case and several short cases will no longer continue. However, the College still recognises the different skills which these two parts of the previous exam assessed, i.e. history taking, communication and management planning were assessed principally by the long case and the ability to elicit physical signs by the short cases. From October 2004, all these skills will be assessed within a single circuit format exam (Fig. 1.1). Communication skills, history taking and management will be assessed over two stations, each of 9 minutes, and one 22-minute station, under direct observation by examiners. The ability to elicit physical signs and interpret them will be assessed by six stations, each of 9 minutes, covering development, neurology, cardiology and three other body systems or skills. Again, these six stations will be directly observed and scored by examiners.

The most difficult part of any clinical examination is the short case. The candidate must decide quickly what is wrong with the child and it is this ability to gently, quickly and correctly elicit physical signs and rapidly interpret them which the short cases are designed to test. The time allotted for short cases in the current exam format is 30 minutes; usually each examiner questions the candidate for 15 minutes while the other examiner marks. In the new format, it will be 9 minutes per short case with 4 minutes between stations to rest. There will be no possibility of prolonging your time at a particular station so this will place added emphasis on swift and efficient examination skills and succinct summarising of the findings. The examiners will have seen the cases before and agreed the physical signs, how difficult they are to elicit and whether it is appropriate to expect a postgraduate paediatric trainee to be able to detect all the signs.

The examiners aim to use the short cases to assess the candidate on several different organ systems in order to detect the candidate with specialist knowledge and experience of, say, cardiology but who lacks breadth of clinical examination skills more generally. In particular, many candidates are

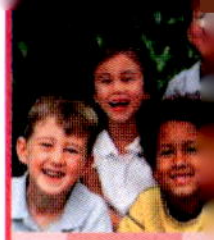

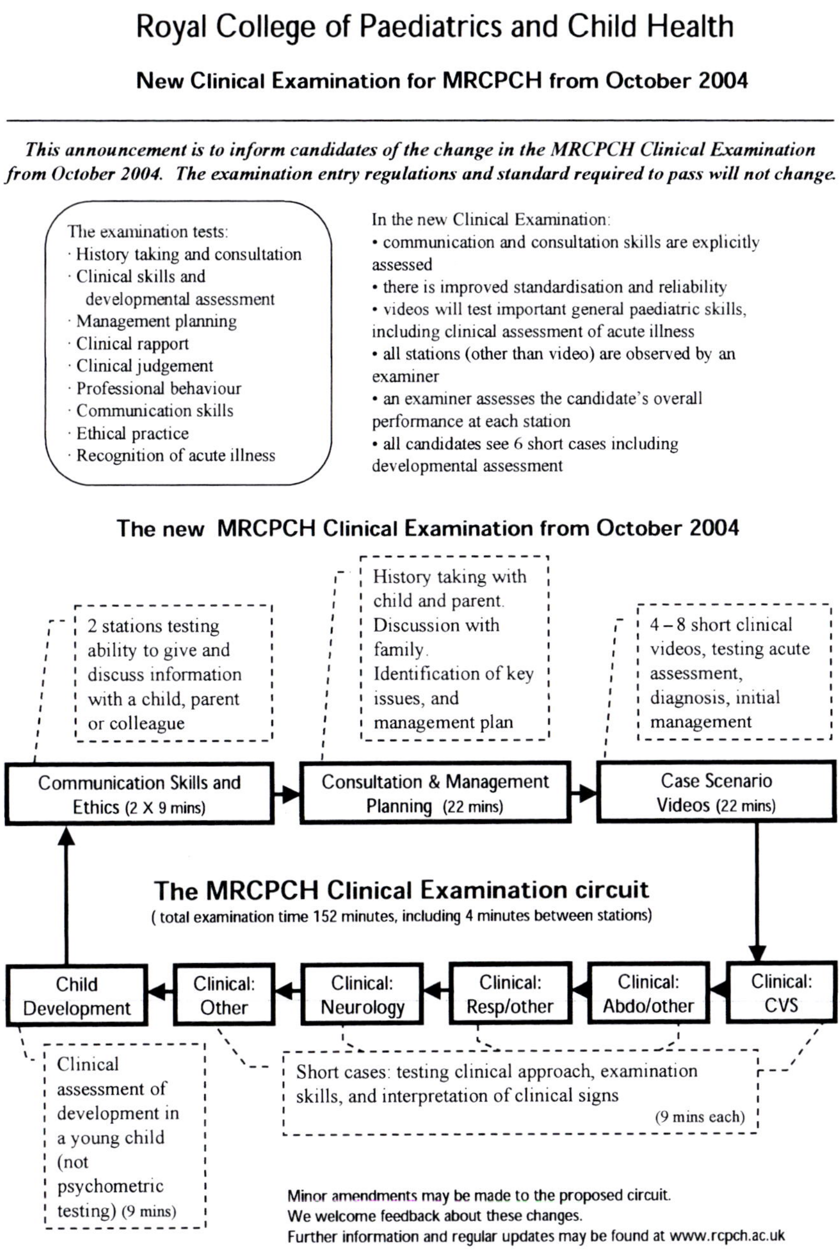
Royal College of Paediatrics and Child Health
New Clinical Examination for MRCPCH from October 2004
This announcement is to inform candidates of the change in the MRCPCH Clinical Examination from October 2004. The examination entry regulations and standard required to pass will not change.
The examination tests:
· History taking and consultation
· Clinical skills and developmental assessment
· Management planning
· Clinical rapport
· Clinical judgement
· Professional behaviour
· Communication skills
· Ethical practice
· Recognition of acute illness
In the new Clinical Examination:
• communication and consultation skills are explicitly assessed
• there is improved standardisation and reliability
• videos will test important general paediatric skills, including clinical assessment of acute illness
• all stations (other than video) are observed by an examiner
• an examiner assesses the candidate's overall performance at each station
• all candidates see 6 short cases including developmental assessment
The new MRCPCH Clinical Examination from October 2004
2 stations testing ability to give and discuss information with a child, parent or colleague
History taking with child and parent. Discussion with family. Identification of key issues, and management plan
4 – 8 short clinical videos, testing acute assessment, diagnosis, initial management
Communication Skills and Ethics (2 X 9 mins)
Consultation & Management Planning (22 mins)
Case Scenario Videos (22 mins)
The MRCPCH Clinical Examination circuit
(total examination time 152 minutes, including 4 minutes between stations)
Child Development
Clinical: Other
Clinical: Neurology
Clinical: Resp/other
Clinical: Abdo/other
Clinical: CVS
Clinical assessment of development in a young child (not psychometric testing) (9 mins)
Short cases: testing clinical approach, examination skills, and interpretation of clinical signs (9 mins each)
Minor amendments may be made to the proposed circuit.
We welcome feedback about these changes.
Further information and regular updates may be found at www.rcpch.ac.uk

Fig. 1.1 *The new MRCPCH clinical examination circuit.*
(Adapted from material on the RCPCH website, www.rcpch.ac.uk, March 2004. Courtesy of the Royal College of Paediatrics and Child Health.)

strong at either developmental examination or at physical examination of hearts, chests and abdomens, but not both. Very few are expert at neurological examination and eye examination seems a recurrent weakness. Currently, MRCPCH examiners aim to assess each candidate on at least four systems, almost always including a developmental assessment. In the new format, all candidates will be examined on six short cases. You may be asked

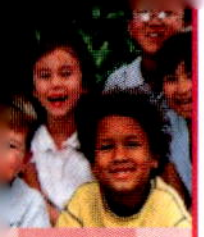

to examine an entirely normal child. Newer techniques involving the use of teaching aids such as cardiopulmonary resuscitation models, videos, etc. may also be used. There will also be four to eight short clinical videos (a separate 22-minute station) to assess 'end of the bed' diagnosis and emergency scenarios which cannot be replicated in an exam setting.

APPROACH TO THE SHORT CASE

Begin each short case by introducing yourself. Try to talk to the child as much as possible. Get down to the child's level and place the child in the position you want. Keep a young child on the parent's lap if possible. This is when a well-rehearsed, swift technique for each system, for syndromes and for developmental assessment will stand you in good stead. Candidates must clean their hands between examining patients.

The examination of a short case is frequently introduced by a piece of history, e.g. the examiner might simply say, 'Look at this child and tell me what you notice', or, alternatively, 'This young girl has become cyanosed over the last few months, why do you think this might be?' The first question is all-embracing. However, examiners are encouraged by the College to introduce the case in order that the examination bears some similarity to real clinical practice, in which a child is rarely examined 'blind' to the history or presentation. The second type of question is therefore an invitation to show that you can examine the relevant parts quickly, as you would have to do in a busy outpatient clinic or emergency department, and step outside the artificial restraints of a single system examination. This difficult skill of 'rationalised examination' presumes as an essential prerequisite that you know the differential diagnosis of common physical signs. For example, if you do not know that the differential of a lump in the neck includes a lymphoma, you will not automatically offer to examine for hepatosplenomegaly and will be marked down compared to a candidate who does and can explain why.

'RATIONALISED EXAMINATION'

Examiners use three common patterns of assessment:

1. Full system examination (e.g. examine the child's cardiovascular system)
2. Specific task (e.g. palpate the child's praecordium and listen to the heart)
3. Simple observation (e.g. observe the child on the parent's knee and tell me what you observe).

The candidate who is given a specific task should perform this. If asked to palpate the abdomen, do not begin by examining the hands. Candidates will *not* be penalised for following instructions. However, after examining the abdomen, always offer to examine other relevant parts. A candidate will not be penalised when a child becomes unhappy or upset during examination provided this is not the result of the candidate's technique.

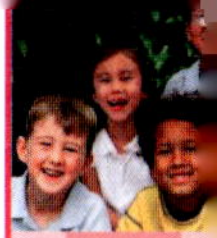

However, the candidate is not expected to give up immediately either. Playful cajoling of the reluctant child or encouraging the shy child are all part of real-life paediatrics. You will fare better if you have some small toys ready to hand to help with distraction and if the tone of your voice and the language you use is age appropriate. Always enlist the parent's help in settling and distracting the child. If the child becomes distraught, however, it is reasonable to ask the examiner whether you should persevere.

Perfect the habit of thinking through the sequence:

1. differential diagnosis
2. examine relevant parts
3. exclude alternative diagnoses
4. final diagnosis

so that this process is second nature even when you are confronted by a situation which we have not covered.

The assessment of a short case by a candidate can be made at three levels.

1. If you are certain of the diagnosis, don't 'beat about the bush' – for example, 'This child has a glycogen storage disease.' This response scores maximum marks if you are right, but if you are wrong you get no marks for 'rough work'.
2. If you are less confident of your diagnosis, an appropriate statement might be: 'The abnormal findings were a very large liver, palpable kidneys, doll's face and short stature. This is consistent with one of the storage diseases due to an inborn error of metabolism.' Even if your interpretation is wrong, you will still gain marks if the physical signs are correct.
3. If you cannot fit the signs together to make a diagnosis, the best approach is to list the important negative and positive findings – for example: 'There is a 10 cm, smooth, non-tender liver and both kidneys are also palpable.' You may then be asked to commit yourself to a diagnosis but this is better than overconfidently plumping for a diagnosis initially when the signs obviously did not fit, especially if it is the wrong diagnosis.

Whichever approach you adopt, you should state the summary of your findings succinctly, clearly and confidently. Many candidates are unsure whether to inform the examiners of physical signs as they elicit them or to wait until they have completed their examination. The examiner may specify whether they want a 'running commentary' or not. If not specified, our advice is to wait until you have completed your examination before informing the examiner of your full findings, except in the case of the developmental examination when it is important to talk as you are going along. In this way we believe you will make fewer errors and will always gain the examiners' full attention.

If you find no abnormalities, say so. Do not invent signs, as sins of commission are worse than sins of omission. Similarly, if you are very uncertain of a physical sign (e.g. whether or not a spleen is palpable), then it is probably not significantly enlarged. Remember, the cases will have been selected on the basis that they have definite physical signs which help the examiners discriminate between good and bad candidates. 'Soft signs' which even the examiners cannot agree on should not result in failure of a candidate. It is better to be confident and say, 'The spleen is not palpable', rather than the oft heard 'I think the spleen may possibly be just palpable'.

For some short cases, you will be asked only the diagnosis and to demonstrate the physical signs. However, some examiners may ask a supplementary question about relevant investigations to confirm the diagnosis, appropriate follow-up, etc.

It is said the more short cases you see in the current format of the MRCPCH, the more likely you are to pass. While it is true that if you are on your sixth case, you are probably doing well, the converse is not true. Some 'short' cases are in fact very complex or involve more than one system and if you have only seen three difficult cases but performed well in all, you are just as likely to pass. Few candidates currently see more than four or five short cases. Each candidate should ideally be examined on every major system of the body (heart, chest, abdomen and a part of the CNS – and many examiners like to see the candidate conduct some aspect of developmental assessment), usually implying a minimum of four cases, unless examination of a particular system has already been covered in the long case. In the latter situation, other systems will be assessed (e.g. skin, locomotor, endocrine). In the new format, all candidates will be assessed on six different systems or skills (e.g. resuscitation skills), ideally in six different children.

Most candidates fail the short cases because of a lack of technique rather than a lack of knowledge. Alternatively, they may fail because of inadequate anticipation of what type of cases to expect. This book should help with both of these pitfalls, but clearly there is no substitute for practising on the wards under exam conditions, with either a fellow candidate or a registrar taking the part of the examiner.

So to sum up, to pass the short cases requires regular practice with an experienced colleague. Short cases which candidates frequently perform poorly on are examination of the eyes, examination of the motor system and developmental examination. It is absolutely essential to develop a professional and thorough system of clinical examination. In paediatrics a child-friendly approach is necessary. A candidate who upsets the patient or parents or is rough in their technique will fail irrespective of their abilities to correctly elicit physical signs. A kind and gentle approach will immediately put the examiners on your side. Do not be afraid to ask the examiner to explain if you are unclear about what is required. Always introduce yourself to the child and parent. Finally, there is no substitute for practice and experience.

Detailed advice on the examination of each system is provided by the complementary publication *Clinical Paediatrics for Postgraduate Examinations 3e* by T Stephenson, H Wallace and A Thomson (Churchill Livingstone, Edinburgh, 2003).

Good luck and enjoy our book.

2 THE CARDIOVASCULAR SYSTEM

The first hurdle in the preparation for the clinical examination is to establish an examination routine for each system that suits you, and to practise it until it is second nature. We provide a checklist for the basic cardiovascular examination below. An in-depth iteration of all the systems examinations is provided in *Clinical Paediatrics for Postgraduate Examinations*, 3rd edition, by T Stephenson, H Wallace and A Thomson (Churchill Livingstone, Edinburgh, 2003).

CARDIOVASCULAR SYSTEM EXAMINATION SUMMARY

INSPECTION

Expose child appropriately and ideally position at 45°.

Whole child General health, nutritional status, dysmorphic features, sweating on forehead

Hands Clubbing, peripheral cyanosis, xanthomas, splinter haemorrhages, absent thumbs, absent radii, abnormal palmar creases

Facies Plethoric, conjunctival injection, pallor, central cyanosis, teeth (conjunctival injection + gum hypertrophy = chronic cyanosis)

Chest Respiratory rate, scars (thoracotomy = operations outside heart, sternotomy = intracardiac), symmetry – look from the side, deformity – Harrison's sulci, visible pulsation

PALPATION

Pulses *Both* brachial, femoral (can do at the end), rate (count for 15 seconds then multiply by 4), quality, rhythm

BP Offer to measure the blood pressure at the end

Apex Locate apex beat (most lateral and inferior impulse) and count ribs to check position, normally fourth intercostal space in midclavicular line, nature of impulse; sustained in AS, forceful in LVH

Praecordium Thrills or heaves, palpable P_2 in pulmonary hypertension

Suprasternal notch Thrill = aortic stenosis

AUSCULTATION

Heart sounds

- Loud S1: ASD, prosthetic valve
- Loud S2: increased pulmonary blood flow (PDA, ASD, VSD), pulmonary hypertension
- Split S2: fixed split (ASD), wide split (ASD, PS, RBBB), reversed split (AS, LBBB)
- Single S2: tetralogy of Fallot, PS
- Extra HS: ejection click (AS/PS), mitral valve prolapse

Murmurs Grade, timing, character, quality, position of maximum intensity, radiation

Back Listen for murmurs and inspiratory crackles if in failure

ANYTHING ELSE?
Blood pressure; femoral pulses; feel for hepatomegaly; plot height and weight on a growth chart appropriate for the child's age and sex

INVESTIGATIONS (which may be appropriate depending on the diagnosis)
Saturation monitor, ABG, ECG, CXR, ECHO, cardiac catheterization

In the exam setting the examiner will give a stem scenario generally followed by one of the following instructions:

- Examine this patient's heart.
- Examine this child's praecordium.
- Feel this child's pulses
- Examine this child's cardiovascular system.
- Look at this child's chest and listen to his heart.

Even when requested to perform a specific task such as feel the pulse or look at the chest, always ensure that you inspect the child for important features outlined in the checklist. Where there is potential for ambiguity in the examiner's request, such as 'examine this child's heart', candidates often debate over whether they should start with examination of the hands. In light of the limited time available and rather than infer your confusion to the examiner, proceed with your examination in the most expedient manner. It takes only a few seconds to inspect the hands and check for finger clubbing and you are unlikely to irritate the examiner in doing so. So much of the examination of the child will require you to be an opportunist in terms of assessment anyway.

CARDIOLOGY SHORT CASES

SMALL VENTRICULAR SEPTAL DEFECT

STEM: This infant had been noted by her family doctor to have a murmur. Please examine her cardiovascular system and tell us what you find.

PRESENTATION OF EXAMINATION FINDINGS

Christine is a well-nourished infant with no dysmorphic features who is not distressed at rest and is pink in air with no finger clubbing. The chest shape is symmetrical with no scars. Her pulse is 140 bpm of normal volume and character and her apex beat is undisplaced. She has a thrill over the lower left sternal edge. The first and second heart sounds are normal. There is a loud grade 4/6 harsh pansystolic murmur present, maximum at the lower left sternal edge which radiates widely throughout the praecordium and through to the back.

Thinking pause.....

These findings are in keeping with a small VSD in an otherwise well child. This is also known as maladie de Roger.

Anything else?

I would like to measure her blood pressure and plot her height and weight on a growth chart appropriate for her age and sex. I would refer Christine to the cardiology team to ensure that she was followed up appropriately.

What advice would you give to the parents?

I would advise good dental hygiene and antibiotic prophylaxis for dental extraction. The parents can be reassured that many septal defects close with time. If it does not close she may still never need surgery; she can lead a full and active life and participate in all sports safely.

LARGE VENTRICULAR SEPTAL DEFECT

STEM: This infant is short of breath at rest and is failing to thrive. Please examine his heart and tell us what you find.

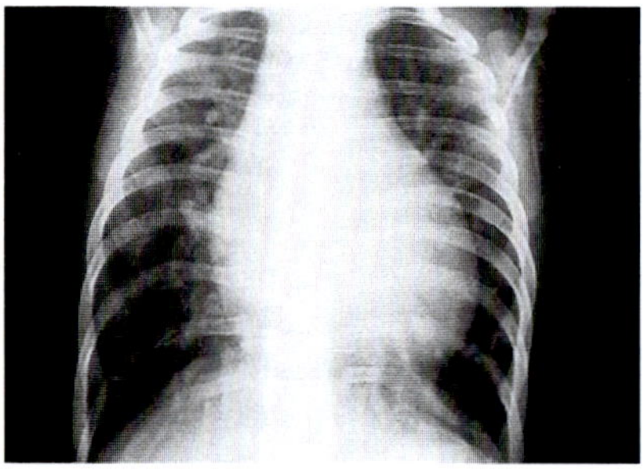

Fig. 2.1 *Chest X-ray showing an enlarged heart in VSD.*
(Reproduced with kind permission from Field D J, Stroobant J (eds) An Illustrated Colour Text: Paediatrics. Edinburgh: Churchill Livingstone, 1997.)

PRESENTATION OF EXAMINATION FINDINGS

Ian is a thin infant with reduced subcutaneous fat. He has no dysmorphic features. He is tachypnoeic at rest with a bulging praecordium more prominent on the left side; Harrison's sulcus is present. His pulse is 140 bpm of normal volume and character. The apex beat is well localised and thrusting, suggesting left ventricular hypertrophy. The first and second heart sounds are present with no added sounds. He has a harsh, loud, 3/6 pansystolic murmur loudest at the lower left sternal edge but widely conducted throughout the praecordium. A soft mid-diastolic murmur can be heard over the apex. His lung bases are clear and there is no hepatomegaly.

Thinking pause.....

These findings are in keeping with a diagnosis of a large ventricular septal defect with evidence of left ventricular hypertrophy and increased blood flow across the mitral valve secondary to the large left to right shunt. He is not in heart failure at present. I would also like to plot his height and weight on a growth chart appropriate for his age and sex.

Anything else?

I would like to take a dietary history, as he appears to be failing to thrive. Drug history is also important as he may already be on a diuretic and ACE inhibitor. Also I would perform an ECG to confirm left ventricular hypertrophy. I would seek a cardiology opinion as he will require echocardiography. Surgical closure of the VSD will be necessary.

When would you consider surgical closure of a VSD?

- Small: regular review (most close spontaneously)
- Moderate: regular review, may require diuretics, surgical closure
- Large: surgical closure <3 months of age to prevent pulmonary hypertension and ensure adequate weight gain.

What do you know about the role of digoxin?

There is evidence to suggest that digoxin has no beneficial effect in the absence of failure and may indeed adversely affect feeding.

Signs of moderate to large VSD

Cardiomegaly, soft systolic murmur, diastolic murmur at apex, plethora. Don't forget Eisenmenger's syndrome, characterised by cyanosis and clubbing due to right to left shunt through the VSD.

ATRIAL SEPTAL DEFECT

STEM: This boy was found to have an incidental murmur during a routine assessment by his family doctor. Please examine his cardiovascular system and tell us what you find.

PRESENTATION OF EXAMINATION FINDINGS

Liam is a happy, well-nourished 5-year-old boy with normal facies. He is pink and has no finger clubbing. His pulse is 120 bpm and both brachial and femoral pulses are of normal volume and character. He has no thrills or heaves and his apex beat is undisplaced. The first and second heart sounds are present and he has fixed splitting of his second heart sound. There is a 2/6 ejection systolic murmur heard loudest over the upper left sternal edge with no radiation to the back.

Thinking pause.....

These findings are in keeping with an ASD. I would also like to measure his blood pressure and plot his height and weight on a growth chart appropriate for his age and sex.

If the examiner asks 'Is the blood pressure ever abnormal with ASD alone?' you should reply that measurement of blood pressure is a routine part of your examination but you would expect it to be normal.

Could this be the murmur of pulmonary stenosis?

The murmur of pulmonary stenosis is heard loudest over this area but generally radiates through to the back and is accompanied by an ejection click and a soft or absent second heart sound. Furthermore there was fixed splitting of the second heart sound in keeping with an ASD.

How would you manage this patient?

Children with ASDs are reviewed regularly. ASDs tend not to close spontaneously and require surgical closure before the age of 5 years to prevent arrhythmias, pulmonary hypertension or reduced exercise tolerance in later life. Closure can be performed safely and successfully during cardiac catheterisation using an Angelwings, Amplatz or Cardioseal device. Studies have shown that correction in the first decade increases life expectancy. The risk of bacterial endocarditis complicating an ASD is very rare but antibiotic prophylaxis should be recommended (see *British National Formulary* guidelines).

PULMONARY STENOSIS

STEM: This boy was noted to have a heart murmur by his school doctor who wanted your assessment to know whether or not it was significant.

PRESENTATION OF EXAMINATION FINDINGS

David is a pleasant, healthy looking 7-year-old boy with no dysmorphic features. He is pink in air with no finger clubbing. Both brachial pulses are present at a rate of 120 bpm regular and of normal character and volume. His femoral pulses are normal. There are no scars and he has a prominent sternum. His apex beat is undisplaced and he has a right ventricular impulse at the left sternal border. The first and second heart sounds are present with a soft pulmonary component and there is an ejection click after the first heart sound. There is a harsh, 3/6 ejection systolic murmur maximum at the upper left sternal edge which radiates through to the back.

Thinking pause.....
These findings would support the diagnosis of pulmonary stenosis.

Anything else?
I would like to perform an ECG to look for right ventricular hypertrophy and a degree of right bundle branch block. A specialist cardiology opinion is required to do an echocardiogram and decide on appropriate management.

What are the indications for intervention?
Balloon dilatation valvoplasty is usually indicated once the gradient across the valve is greater than 40 mmHg or the right ventricular pressure is greater than 60 mmHg.

AORTIC STENOSIS

STEM: This 6-year-old girl has been noted to have a heart murmur by her GP. Please examine her heart and tell us what you find.

PRESENTATION OF EXAMINATION FINDINGS

Rachel is a pink, well-nourished 6-year-old girl who is undistressed at rest, with no finger clubbing. Her pulse is 100 bpm and slow rising. The apex beat is undisplaced but is forceful in nature. She has a soft, systolic thrill palpable in the suprasternal notch and a slow rising carotid pulse. The first and second heart sounds are present and an early systolic ejection click can be heard over the apex. There is a 4/6 ejection systolic murmur loudest at the right upper sternal edge radiating up to the carotids. The femoral pulses are normal.

Thinking pause.....
These findings are consistent with a diagnosis of aortic stenosis. I would like to measure the blood pressure and in particular I would be looking for a narrow pulse pressure. I would also like to plot her height and weight on a growth chart appropriate for her age and sex.

How would you manage this patient?
I would like to do a chest X-ray to look for cardiomegaly and poststenotic dilatation. An ECG may confirm left ventricular hypertrophy but does not accurately reflect the degree of stenosis. Echocardiogram and Doppler studies are important to determine the gradient across the aortic valve. It may be possible at this point to perform balloon dilatation of the valve, although there is the risk of aortic regurgitation associated with this. For re-stenosis or critical aortic stenosis, surgical replacement of the aortic valve is required.

What advice would you give to the parents?
If the gradient across the valve is more than 50 mmHg I would advise the parents that Rachel must not participate in strenuous sports. I would emphasise the need for good dental hygiene and mandatory requirement for prophylactic antibiotics during dental extraction.

COARCTATION OF AORTA

STEM: This 8-year-old boy is due for circumcision under general anaesthetic. The anaesthetist has examined him and cannot feel his femoral pulse. Please can you examine his cardiovascular system and present your findings.

PRESENTATION OF EXAMINATION FINDINGS

Daniel is a well looking 8-year-old boy who is not cyanosed and does not have finger clubbing. His pulse is 100 bpm and both brachial pulses are present; however, his femoral pulses are absent. He has a forceful apex beat which is undisplaced and he has no thrills or heaves. The first and second heart sounds are normal and there is a 3/6 ejection systolic murmur at the upper left sternal edge radiating through to the back between the scapulae.

Thinking pause.....
These findings are in keeping with a diagnosis of coarctation of the aorta. I would like to measure his blood pressure and record his height and weight on a growth chart. As Daniel is 8 years old I would like to see a chest X-ray to look for evidence of rib notching as evidence of the presence of collateral vessels.

As most coarctations are picked up at a younger age prior to the development of collaterals, how would you now manage this boy?
Doppler studies or cardiac catheterisation is required to measure the degree of stenosis. It is most likely that he will require cardiac surgery to repair the coarctation, either by excision of the stenotic area and end–end anastomosis, or by a left subclavian flap. Balloon dilatation is an alternative, although less successful, option and may be associated with re-coarctation or development of an aortic aneurysm.

TETRALOGY OF FALLOT

STEM: Melanie had spells of going blue as a small baby. Please examine her cardiovascular system and tell us what you find.

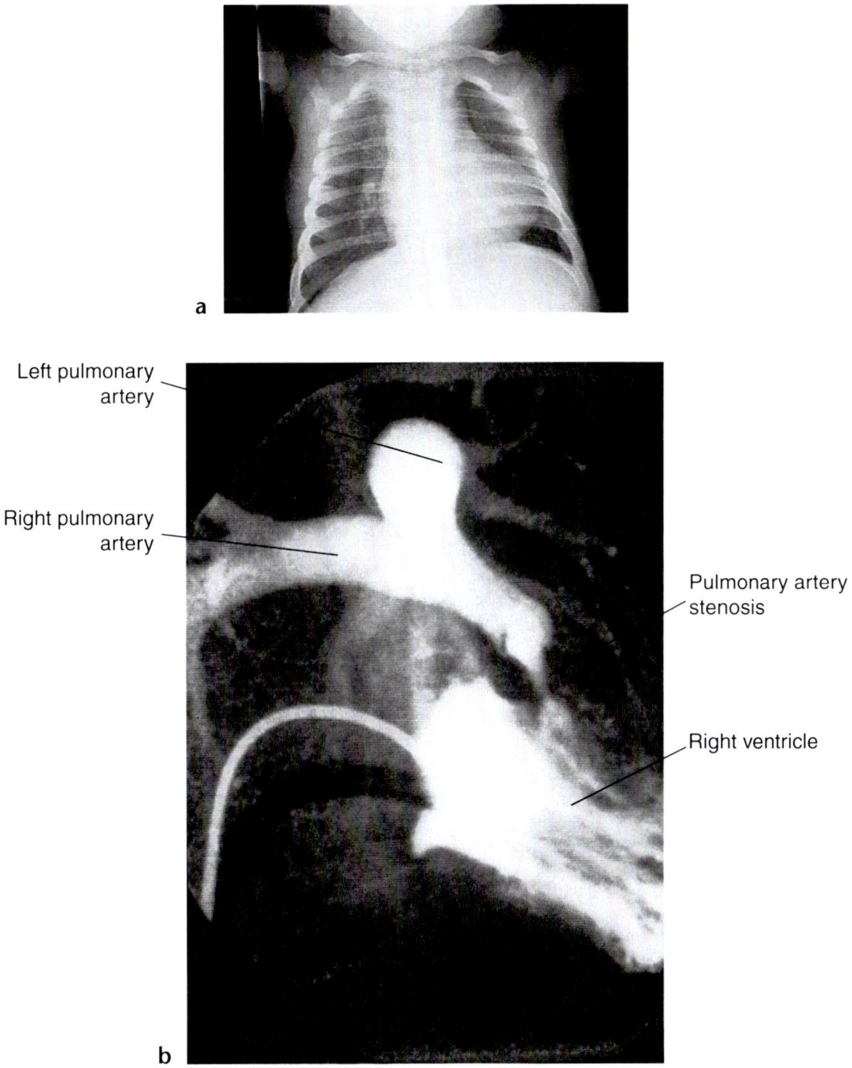

Fig. 2.2 (**a**) *Chest X-ray in tetralogy of Fallot;* (**b**) *angiogram of tetralogy of Fallot.* (Reproduced with kind permission from Field D J, Stroobant J (eds) An Illustrated Colour Text: Paediatrics. Edinburgh: Churchill Livingstone, 1997.)

PRESENTATION OF EXAMINATION FINDINGS

Melanie is an infant with no dysmorphic features who is thin with reduced subcutaneous tissue. She has a plethoric face with conjunctival injection and central cyanosis. Her pulse is 120 bpm and of normal volume. Both brachial pulses are present and her femoral pulses are normal with no brachiofemoral delay. Melanie has a right thoracotomy scar and a prominent sternum. Her apex beat is undisplaced and she has a single second heart sound. There is a 3/6 ejection systolic murmur at the upper left sternal edge and a 3/6 continuous murmur below the right clavicle.

Thinking pause.....

These findings are in keeping with a diagnosis of tetralogy of Fallot with a right modified Blalock–Taussig shunt. I would like to measure her blood pressure and plot her height and weight on a growth chart appropriate for her age and sex.

Why did you say a modified BT-shunt?

If a classical Blalock–Taussig shunt is performed the brachial pulse is absent, unlike a modified shunt where the pulse is generally still palpable, as in this case.

How would you manage this patient?

Surgery is the definitive treatment for tetralogy of Fallot. Without treatment 85% of these children will die by their second decade. Appropriate medical management prior to surgery is necessary. There are three very important areas of management:

1. Monitoring of the haematocrit (aim to keep it below 60%) as increased viscosity is associated with cerebrovascular events. Cerebrovascular accidents can also occur with relative anaemia, the most likely cause of which would be due to iron deficiency and the child should be treated appropriately. Coagulation should be monitored as coagulation deficiencies are more common in those with a high haematocrit.
2. Antibiotic prophylaxis for dental treatment is mandatory as tetralogy of Fallot is particularly associated with infective endocarditis.
3. Hypercyanotic spells are common in infants and they will often adopt a squatting position to help relieve episodes of increased cyanosis by increasing the systemic resistance and consequently increasing pulmonary blood flow. Although the majority of these 'hypoxic spells' are self-limiting they can be fatal. Treatment involves administering 100% oxygen, with the child in the knee–elbow position, and propranolol (peripheral vasoconstriction and reduced pulmonary muscular spasm). Morphine sedation and pain relief may be required and if very severe, artificial ventilation and potent peripheral vasoconstrictors (e.g. noradrenaline).

WILLIAMS' SYNDROME

STEM: This engaging and chatty 6-year-old girl attends a school for children with special needs and has been noted to have a heart murmur by the school doctor. Please examine her and tell us what you find.

PRESENTATION OF EXAMINATION FINDINGS

Hollie is a chatty 6-year-old girl with prominent lips, short palpebral fissures, stellate irises and medial eyebrow flare. She also has a relatively small chin

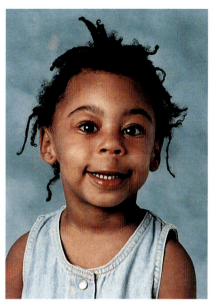

Fig. 2.3 *Facial dysmorphism in Williams' syndrome.*
(Reproduced with kind permission from Field D J, Stroobant J (eds) An Illustrated Colour Text: Paediatrics. Edinburgh: Churchill Livingstone, 1997.)

with small teeth. Her nails are hypoplastic but there is no clubbing and she is pink. Her pulse is 90 bpm and is regular and of normal volume. Her apex beat is undisplaced. She has a thrill in the suprasternal notch. The first and second heart sounds are normal and there is no ejection click. She has a 4/6 ejection systolic murmur loudest over the right upper sternal edge and radiating up to the carotids.

Thinking pause.....

Hollie is a girl with Williams' syndrome and aortic valve stenosis, most likely to be supravalvular in nature.

Anything else?

I would like to measure her blood pressure and listen for renal bruits as these children can have renal artery stenosis (middle aorta syndrome). I would also like to plot her height, weight and head circumference on a growth chart appropriate for her age and sex.

Would you like to ask the parents any questions?

'Did Hollie have any problems in the newborn period with too much calcium in her body?' 'Does she receive additional help at school?'

How would you confirm you diagnosis?

FISH studies looking for a microdeletion on chromosome 7 to confirm Williams' syndrome and cardiac catheterisation to assess the degree of aortic stenosis.

Features of Williams' syndrome

Features of Williams' syndrome are outlined in Box 2.1.

Box 2.1 Features of Williams' syndrome

Face	■ Prominent lips, open mouth ■ Medial eyebrow flare ■ Short palpebral fissures ■ Blue eyes, stellate calcification of the iris
CVS	■ Supravalvular aortic stenosis ■ Less commonly valvular AS, PS, peripheral PS
CNS	■ Mild microcephaly ■ Learning difficulties (average IQ 56)
Skeletal	■ Mild IUGR ■ Hypoplastic nails
Others	■ Bladder diverticula ■ Renal artery stenosis

NOONAN'S SYNDROME

STEM: This short boy was referred by the community paediatrician for assessment of his dysmorphic features and heart murmur. Please examine him and present your findings.

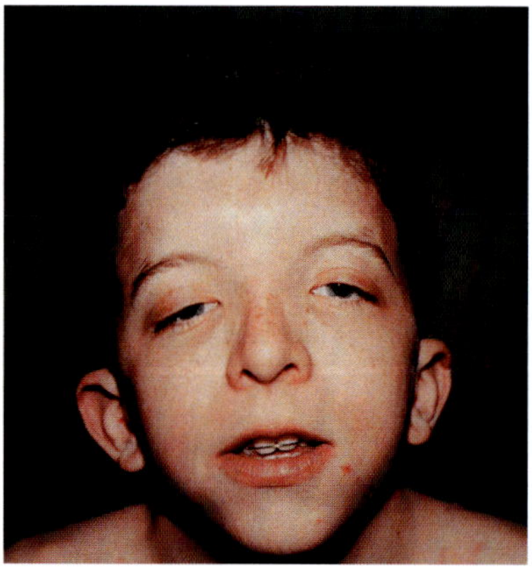

Fig. 2.4 *Facial phenotype in Noonan's syndrome.*
(Reproduced with kind permission from Lissauer T, Clayden G. Illustrated Textbook of Paediatrics, 2nd edn. Edinburgh: Mosby, 2001.)

PRESENTATION OF EXAMINATION FINDINGS

Philip is an 8-year-old boy with a broad forehead with hypertelorism, downward sloping palpebral fissures, epicanthic folds and partial bilateral ptosis. He has webbing of the neck with a low posterior hairline. He has micrognathia and a high arched palate. He appears to be of short stature, although I would like to plot him on a growth chart, and he has cubitus valgus. His chest is shield shaped with widely spaced nipples and pectus excavatum. Philip is pink in air with no finger clubbing. His pulse is 110 bpm and of normal volume and character. His apex beat is undisplaced and he has a parasternal heave. The first and second heart sounds are present with a widely split second heart sound and an ejection click. He has a 3/6 ejection systolic murmur heard loudest over the upper left sternal edge and radiating through to the back.

Thinking pause.....

This is a young boy with Noonan's syndrome who has pulmonary valve stenosis. I would also like to measure his blood pressure and plot his height and weight on a growth chart appropriate for his age and sex.

What is Noonan's syndrome?

This is an autosomal dominantly inherited condition, but with variable phenotypic expression between generations, occurring in approximately 1 in 2000 of the population. It is associated with a defect on chromosome 12. Noonan's syndrome is a collection of features as outlined above and includes other signs such as kyphoscoliosis, kyphosis, small penis, cryptorchidism, renal anomalies, bleeding problems and reduced IQ.

What cardiac anomalies are associated with it?

These children may have pulmonary valve stenosis, peripheral pulmonary stenosis, ASD and cardiomyopathy. This boy has pulmonary valve stenosis as I could hear an ejection click.

How do the cardiac anomalies differ from Turner's syndrome?

Turner's syndrome is generally associated with coarctation of the aorta, aortic stenosis and bicuspid aortic valve.

DOWN'S SYNDROME

STEM: This baby girl has been referred because of feeding difficulties. Please could you do a general assessment and examine her cardiovascular system and tell us what you find.

PRESENTATION OF EXAMINATION FINDINGS

Harriet is a small, thin, 10-month-old child with features consistent with Down's syndrome. She is centrally cyanosed and has finger clubbing but is otherwise undistressed with no signs of heart failure. Her pulse is 120 bpm of normal character and volume. She has a prominent sternum with visible cardiac pulsation. Her apex beat is forceful and displaced to the fifth intercostal space in the anterior axillary line. She also has a parasternal heave. The first and second heart sounds are present and there is a loud, harsh 3/6 pansystolic murmur maximal at the lower left sternal edge conducted throughout the praecordium. There is also a soft mid-diastolic murmur at the lower left sternal edge. The lung bases are clear and there is no hepatomegaly.

Thinking pause.....
In summary this is an infant with Down's syndrome and the most likely cardiac anomaly is atrioventricular septal defect.

Anything else?
I would like to plot her height and weight on a growth chart appropriate for her age and sex. I would like to do a chest X-ray and ECG to look for cardiomegaly and confirm biventricular hypertrophy. Echocardiography is the best investigation to fully assess the anatomy, although cardiac catheterisation will be required to assess the degree of pulmonary hypertension.

When would you repair the defect?
Generally speaking, complete atrioventricular septal defects require early repair before the age of 2 years to prevent the development of pulmonary hypertension with consequent pulmonary vascular disease. For partial defects surgery is usually carried out between the ages of 2 and 5 years. In children with Down's syndrome the repair is usually earlier as they have an increased propensity to develop pulmonary vascular disease.

INNOCENT MURMUR

STEM: Louise was noted to have a murmur by her family doctor during her routine developmental assessment. Do you think this is significant?

PRESENTATION OF EXAMINATION FINDINGS

Louise is a well-nourished 3-year-old girl who is undistressed at rest, pink in air, with no dysmorphic features. Her pulse is 105 bpm of normal volume and character. Her apex beat is undisplaced and both heart sounds are present and normally split. She has a 2/6 systolic murmur at the lower left sternal edge with no radiation. The intensity of the murmur reduces on lying supine. Her femoral pulses are normal. I would like to measure her blood pressure and plot her height and weight on a growth chart appropriate for her age and sex.

Thinking pause.....
This murmur is most likely to be an innocent murmur which is not significant.

Why do you say it is an 'innocent' murmur?

This murmur fulfils the criteria for an innocent murmur, i.e. it is a soft, short systolic murmur, covering a small area, in a symptom-free child. The murmur is affected by posture (sitting/standing). The chest shape is normal and there is normal splitting of the second heart sound. There are no other abnormal signs. I would expect the ECG and chest X-ray to be normal, although they are probably not indicated in this case. However, an innocent murmur can be difficult to distinguish from a small VSD and if I were in any doubt I would request the opinion of a cardiologist for Louise.

What advice would you give the parents?

I would explain that innocent murmurs are very common in young children, occurring in about 50% of under-5 year olds. A murmur is the noise of blood flowing through the heart and it does not compromise the child's well-being. I would reassure the parents that Louise does not require any restriction to her lifestyle.

CYANOSIS

STEM: This boy has been under the care of the general paediatrician with a heart murmur. However, he has been lost to follow-up until recently. Please examine his cardiovascular system and present your findings.

PRESENTATION OF EXAMINATION FINDINGS

Ross is a 14-year-old boy with normal facies who is cyanosed at rest, with no signs of respiratory distress. He is clubbed and has normal pulses. His apex beat is displaced to the fifth intercostal space in the anterior axillary line and he has a left parasternal heave. On auscultation he has a loud pulmonary component of the second heart sound. He has a 2/6 systolic murmur heard over the upper left sternal edge and a diastolic murmur heard along the left sternal edge. There is also a soft pansystolic murmur heard at the lower left sternal edge.

Thinking pause.....
Ross is a boy with a VSD and biventricular hypertrophy and evidence of pulmonary hypertension which is now irreversible and has resulted in Eisenmenger's syndrome.

What is cyanosis?

Cyanosis is a bluish discoloration to the skin or mucous membranes, easily detectable when there is more than 5 g/dl of deoxygenated blood in the skin capillaries. It can be peripheral, due to poor perfusion of the vessels, or central, due to a reduction in the oxygen saturation of arterial blood, usually less than 75% for a haemoglobin of 12–16 g/dl. Therefore cyanosis may be present at a normal PaO_2 if there is polycythemia or not detectable if there is concomitant anaemia. Very occasionally cyanosis is due to the presence of the abnormal pigments sulphaemoglobin or methaemoglobin in the bloodstream, confirmed by spectroscopic examination of the blood. The oxygen arterial tension is normal.

SCARS

STEM: This boy has undergone several heart operations. Please examine his cardiovascular system and tell us what you find.

PRESENTATION OF EXAMINATION FINDINGS

Cameron is a 5-year-old boy with no dysmorphic features but of a slim build and reduced subcutaneous tissue. He is cyanosed at rest with finger clubbing. On inspection of his chest he has a prominent sternum with a midline sternotomy scar and three small scars in the epigastric area. Cameron also has right and left lateral thoracotomy scars. His pulse is 110 bpm and regular and both brachial pulses are present. His apex is displaced to the fifth intercostal space and is forceful in nature. He also has a left parasternal heave. On auscultation the first and second heart sounds are heard and there is a 3/6 continuous murmur loudest at the upper sternal edges but radiating throughout the chest. He also has an elevated JVP, crackles at both lung bases and a 4 cm hepatomegaly and sacral oedema.

Thinking pause.....

In summary this is a young boy with complex cyanotic congenital heart disease who has undergone a number of surgical procedures, which are likely to include pulmonary artery banding or modified shunting and major intracardiac surgery. The epigastric scars may be secondary to pericardial drains or temporary postoperative cardiac pacing. Cameron has clinical evidence of biventricular hypertrophy and a degree of right and left heart failure.

Anything else?

I would like to measure his blood pressure and plot his height and weight on a growth chart appropriate for his age and sex. I would also like to do a chest X-ray to look for pulmonary oedema, and an ECG to confirm biventricular hypertrophy. To assess the degree of ventricular dilatation and valve competence I would ask for a cardiology opinion and to perform an echocardiogram.

How would you manage this patient?

This involves management of the short-term problems with consideration of the longer term prognosis. Initial management requires treating his cardiac failure and optimizing his cardiac output. This can be achieved by a combination of fluid restriction and medication. A combination of diuretics and ACE inhibitors would be first line. Potassium-sparing diuretics should be used with loop diuretics to avoid hyperkalaemia. Cardiac glycosides can also be used with some effect in combination with ACE inhibitors and diuretics. In patients already taking high-dose loop diuretics, ACE inhibitors must be introduced with caution to avoid profound hypotension. The longer term management of Cameron will be the remit of the cardiology team and requires an understanding of his complex cardiac disease and whether further surgery is feasible or if he requires a combined heart and lung transplant.

Surgical scars

There are a number of reasons for cardiovascular surgical scars on the chest, examples of which are outlined in Table 2.1.

Table 2.1 Surgical scars on the chest

Scar	Operation	Reason for operation and type
Right lateral thoracotomy	BT shunt	Cyanosis + continuous murmur Absent brachial pulse = classical shunt Brachial pulse present = modified shunt
Left lateral thoracotomy	BT shunt Coarctation PA banding PDA	As above ± left brachial pulse Complex CHD ± cyanosis No signs post ligation
Median sternotomy	Intracardiac operation	Various, e.g. bypass surgery, valve surgery

DEXTROCARDIA

STEM: Alastair was admitted with a self-limiting diarrhoeal illness and the junior doctor found it difficult to hear his heart sounds. Please examine his heart and tell us what you find.

PRESENTATION OF EXAMINATION FINDINGS

Alastair is a thin 3-year-old boy with no dysmorphic features. He is pink in air and not distressed at rest. His pulse is 100 bpm of normal volume and character. He has dextrocardia with his apex beat most prominent in the right fourth intercostal space in the midclavicular line. His heart sounds are normal with no murmurs.

Thinking pause.....
I would like to examine his abdomen for situs inversus and to ask the parents for a history of frequent chest infections to support a diagnosis of Kartagener's syndrome.

Why do such children have frequent chest infections?
Dextrocardia is associated with primary ciliary dyskinesia and nasal polyps and as a result these children get frequent respiratory tract infections and sinusitis.

How would you diagnose dextrocardia?
Nasociliary brushings can be taken to look at the function of the cilia and then studied under electron microscopy to look at the ultrastructure. The underlying structural abnormality is absent dynein arms on the cilia, which renders them dysfunctional. Mucociliary clearance can be assessed in a cooperative child by ascertaining the time to taste perception of a saccharin particle placed on the inferior nasal turbinate.

SYNDROMES ASSOCIATED WITH CARDIOVASCULAR LESIONS

Syndromes associated with cardiovascular lesions are outlined in Box 2.2.

Box 2.2 Syndromes associated with cardiovascular lesions

- Down's syndrome: AVSD, VSD, PDA, tetralogy of Fallot
- Turner's syndrome: coarctation, AS, bicuspid aortic valve
- Noonan's syndrome: pulmonary stenosis, peripheral PS, ASD, cardiomyopathy
- Williams' syndrome: supravalvular aortic stenosis, peripheral PS, PS
- Congenital rubella syndrome: PDA, VSD, peripheral PS
- Ellis van Creveld syndrome: ASD
- Holt–Oram syndrome: ASD, VSD
- Maternal SLE: congenital heart block
- Pompe's/Friedreich's ataxia: HOCM
- Ehlers–Danlos syndrome: mitral valve prolapse, tricuspid valve prolapse
- Alagille syndrome: pulmonary stenosis
- Marfan's syndrome: prolapsed mitral valve, aortic valve incompetence, dissecting aortic aneurysm

3
THE RESPIRATORY SYSTEM

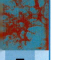

You will be expected to perform an examination of, or part of, the respiratory system and you must have a well-rehearsed routine. A checklist is outlined below.

RESPIRATORY SYSTEM EXAMINATION SUMMARY

INSPECTION (Examine the child on parent's knee if possible)
General well-being, nutritional status, dysmorphic features

Assess
- Respiratory rate
- Colour
- Nasal flaring, recession, accessory muscles
- Stridor, wheeze

Hands Clubbing

Face Cyanosis, traumatic petechiae (coughing)

Neck Tracheal tug

Chest Deformity, scoliosis, Harrison's sulci, hyperinflation

Extras Oxygen, saturation monitors, inhalers, sputum pots, peak flow meters

PALPATION
- Lymphadenopathy (neck and axillae) – can be done at the end
- Feel for apex and trachea
- Expansion

PERCUSSION (not in infant)
- Compare both sides
- Liver (normal position – upper border of the sixth intercostal space)

AUSCULTATION
- 'I'm going to listen to your tummy.'
- Breath sounds: vesicular, bronchial
- Added sounds: crackles, wheeze
- Vocal resonance

ANYTHING ELSE?
- Liver – upper and lower borders
- Measure PEFR: average PEFR in litres/min = (5 times height in cm) – 400; third centile = average PEFR – 50
- Check sputum pot, ENT examination
- Plot height and weight on a growth chart appropriate for age and sex

CYSTIC FIBROSIS

STEM: This young boy has been short of breath for many years. Please examine his chest and tell us what you find.

PRESENTATION OF EXAMINATION FINDINGS

Kenneth is a thin 14-year-old boy with reduced subcutaneous tissues. He is pink in air and undistressed at rest. He has finger clubbing. His chest is hyperinflated and he has an indwelling central venous access device. There is no mediastinal deviation but there is reduced chest expansion on the left side. His chest is dull at the left base with reduced breath sounds and increased vocal resonance. There is a 2 cm liver edge palpable but the liver is displaced downwards due to the hyperinflation of the chest. There are no signs of chronic liver disease.

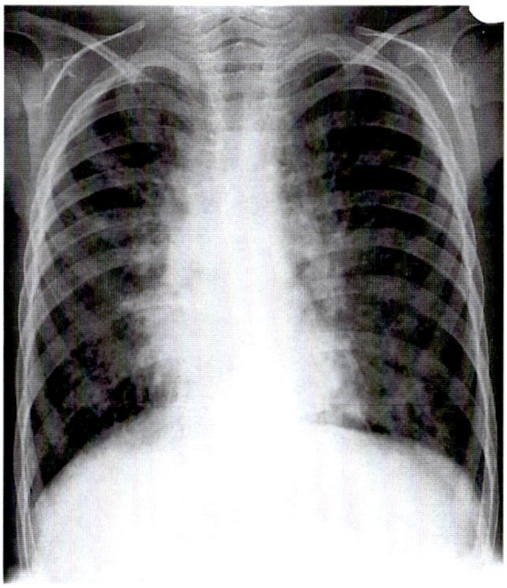

Fig. 3.1 *Chest X-ray in cystic fibrosis showing hyperexpansion, marked peribronchial shadowing, bronchial wall thickening and ring shadows.*
(Reproduced with kind permission from Lissauer T, Clayden G. Illustrated Textbook of Paediatrics, 2nd edn. Edinburgh: Mosby, 2001.)

Thinking pause.....
This is a young boy with cystic fibrosis who has an indwelling central venous access device for frequent courses of antibiotics. He currently has a left lower lobe consolidation.

Anything else?

I would like to plot his height and weight on a growth chart appropriate for his age and sex. I would measure his PEFR and do a chest X-ray to confirm the pneumonia and to radiologically grade his lung disease according to the Chrispen and Norman scoring system: scores of more than 20 indicate advanced disease. It is also important to take a dietary history to ensure that he is taking sufficient calories.

How would you manage this patient?

The immediate management involves treatment of the infection with the appropriate intravenous antibiotics, to which the probable pathogens are sensitive, and daily intense physiotherapy. While he is in hospital it provides us with an opportunity to review his medications and assess his nutritional status.

What can you tell me about the genetics of cystic fibrosis?

Cystic fibrosis is the most common fatal inherited condition in Caucasians. It is an autosomal recessive disease with a carrier rate of 1 in 20 and an incidence of 1 in 2000. It is a multisystem disorder characterised by dysfunction of the exocrine glands resulting in chronic suppurative lung disease, malabsorption, liver disease and infertility. The cystic fibrosis gene is located on the long arm of chromosome 7. Although there are over 700 mutations described in this long 250 kb gene, ΔF508 (deletion of a single phenylalanine residue at amino acid 508) accounts for 78% of mutations in the UK. This gene codes for the protein cystic fibrosis transmembrane regulator (CFTR) which acts as an energy-dependent cyclic AMP-mediated chloride channel blocker. Once the gene has been identified antenatal diagnosis and carrier detection can be performed.

How is CF diagnosed?

Presentation can occur at different ages. A child may present with malabsorption and failure to thrive (30%) and recurrent chest infections (50%) in infancy, although 10% present in the neonatal period with meconium ileus, often associated with microcolon. Various tests are used to assist diagnosis including immunoreactive trypsin, nasal potential differences, gene testing but the definitive diagnosis is made on sweat testing.

Cases can also be identified by prenatal diagnosis or screening. Carrier screening is offered in some centres to mothers at the time of booking. This can be done by either mouth wash or venepuncture and looks for the commonest mutations with a detection rate >85%. Fathers of carrier mothers are then screened followed by amniocentesis or chorionic villus sampling for couples who are both carriers. Termination is offered if the foetus is affected. Neonatal screening is also performed in some centres, by measuring immunoreactive trypsin on the heel prick Guthrie card followed by more definitive testing on positive samples.

How is a sweat test done?

Sweat is collected by pilocarpine iontophoresis either onto filter paper (Gibson and Cook) or in a capillary tube (Wiscor). A minimum of 100 mg of sweat is collected. Sweat sodium of greater than 70 mmol on two occasions is positive. Sweat chloride is greater than sodium, the reverse of normal.

What is the current treatment?

This consists of a multidisciplinary approach with the aim of preventing progression of lung disease and maintaining adequate nutrition and growth. Treatment includes the following:

- Respiratory management
  - physiotherapy × 2–4 per day: chest percussion and postural drainage
  - physical exercise: to strengthen muscles and prevent reaccumulation of secretions
  - prompt treatment of infections
  - prophylaxis: inhaled or oral antibiotics
  - nebulised DNAse, inhaled bronchodilators and inhaled steroids
- Nutrition
  - pancreatic supplements
  - antacids, proton pump inhibitors to enhance small bowel alkalinity so that pancreatic enzyme supplements work better
  - vitamin supplements
  - high calorie diet
  - monitor for liver disease
- Psychological
  - patient and family
- Lung transplant
  - may be indicated in advanced disease

CLUBBING

STEM: This young girl has a chronic cough. Please examine her respiratory system and tell us what you find.

PRESENTATION OF EXAMINATION FINDINGS

Ellie is a slim 8-year-old girl who has finger clubbing. She has no dysmorphic features, no cyanosis or respiratory distress at rest and no evidence of chronic liver disease. She has no chest scars although her chest is hyperinflated. On auscultation she has a few scattered coarse crackles and occasional expiratory wheeze. She also has an empty sputum pot by her bedside. Her heart sounds are normal and she has no murmurs.

Thinking pause.....

Ellie is a young girl with finger clubbing most likely associated with cystic fibrosis.

What conditions is finger clubbing associated with?

Conditions associated with finger clubbing are outlined in Box 3.1. The commonest causes in exams, in descending order, are: cystic fibrosis, Kartagener's syndrome, cyanotic heart disease and IBD.

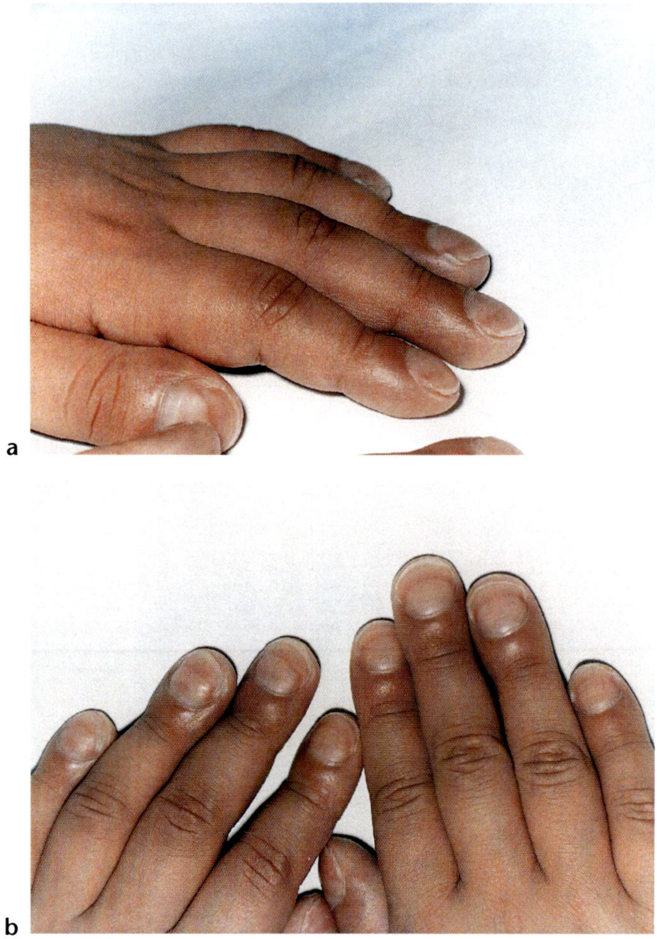

Fig. 3.2 (**a**, **b**) *Finger clubbing and thickening of the proximal interphalanges of hypertrophic pulmonary osteoarthropathy.*

BRONCHIECTASIS

> **STEM:** This boy is short of breath and has a chronic productive cough. Please examine his chest and tell us what you find.

PRESENTATION OF EXAMINATION FINDINGS

Keith is a thin teenage boy who is mildly cyanosed, with halitosis and has finger clubbing. His chest is barrel shaped with a prominent sternum and Harrison's sulcus. He is tachypnoeic at rest with a respiratory rate of 30 breaths per minute and he is using his intercostal muscles. Keith's apex beat is on the left side and is undisplaced. His chest is dull to percussion at both

Box 3.1 Conditions associated with finger clubbing

Respiratory system

- Cystic fibrosis
- Bronchiectasis
- Abscess/empyema
- Fibrosing alveolitis

Cardiovascular system

- Cyanotic congenital heart disease
- Bacterial endocarditis
- AV fistula
- Atrial myxoma

Gastrointestinal system

- Crohn's/UC
- GI lymphoma
- Cirrhosis

Others

- Familial thyrotoxicosis – thyroid acropachy

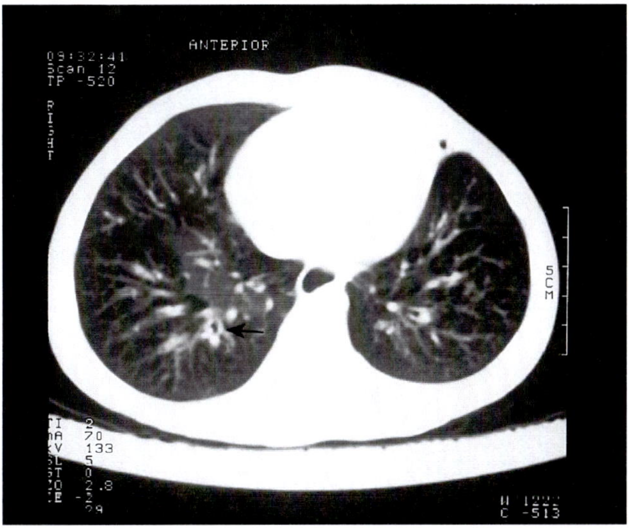

Fig. 3.3 *CT scan of bronchiectasis. The arrow indicates an enlarged airway with surrounding inflammation.*
(Reproduced with kind permission from Field D J, Stroobant J (eds) An Illustrated Colour Text: Paediatrics. Edinburgh: Churchill Livingstone, 1997.)

bases. He has reduced air entry with coarse inspiratory crepitations at both bases. Vocal resonance is also reduced.

Thinking pause.....
This is a boy with probable cystic fibrosis with acquired bronchiectasis.

What other causes do you know of bronchiectasis?

- Immunodeficiencies*
- Kartagener's syndrome*
- Post infection (rare in UK): measles, pertussis
- Foreign body
- Tracheobronchomalacia
- Lobar sequestration
- Alpha-1-antitrypsin deficiency
- Rare syndromes: Macleod's, Klinefelter's, Gardner's

**Currently commonest causes in UK.*

What are the general principles of management of bronchiectasis?

This would include management of any identifiable underlying disorder, physiotherapy and prompt antibiotics during infective episodes. If the disease process is localised and the remaining lung has relatively good function then lobectomy of the affected area is possible.

Where is the commonest site for lobectomy?

The left lower lobe has the poorest drainage and is the most vulnerable to the changes of bronchiectasis. If bronchiectasis is secondary to foreign body aspiration then the right middle lobe will be the most commonly affected area.

CHRONIC STRIDOR

STEM: This baby has difficulty breathing. It tends to be worse when she is crying. Please examine her chest and present your findings.

PRESENTATION OF EXAMINATION FINDINGS

Tracy is a well-looking, 3-month-old infant with inspiratory stridor present at rest but more pronounced when she is crying. She is pink in air with no evidence of respiratory distress and her chest is clear on auscultation. Her pulse is normal and apex beat is undisplaced. Both heart sounds are present with no murmurs.

Thinking pause.....

As Tracy is well, and does not look like an ex-prem baby, the most likely cause of her stridor is laryngomalacia. I would, however, like to know if the stridor has been present from the first few days after birth and whether Tracy required a period of intubation at birth.

Why do you mention prematurity?

Subglottic stenosis is relatively common in ex-prems, and does not necessarily require long periods of ventilation.

Anything else?

Stridor can result from vascular rings, either in isolation or associated with other congenital cardiac lesions. In such cases the child usually presents with failure to thrive as the vascular ring also causes compression of the oesophagus. Laryngeal nerve palsies also cause stridor from birth but can follow cardiac surgery. When present from birth it may result from a difficult labour requiring forceps causing lateral neck traction. Although very rare, if there is bilateral laryngeal nerve palsy, it can be associated with Arnold–Chiari syndrome. Congenital stridor may arise from laryngeal webs or clefts and from cavernous haemangioma.

What advice would you give to the parents?

This presentation, if present from birth, is characteristic of laryngomalacia and requires no further intervention. I would reassure the parents that the noise is caused by a 'floppy' larynx and will generally resolve by the end of the first year of life as the larynx gets stronger. I would also explain that the stridor will get worse when the baby is agitated or has an upper respiratory tract infection.

How would you manage this patient?

It is unnecessary to perform bronchoscopy in every infant with a confident clinical diagnosis of laryngomalacia, as the risks of general anaesthetic, bronchoscopy/endoscopy and recovery far outweigh the risks of sudden death in children with reported 'benign laryngomalacia'. Bronchoscopy should be reserved for those:

- with stridor persisting beyond 18 months
- where the diagnosis may be in doubt
- with failure to thrive
- with apnoeic or cyanotic episodes.

CHRONIC LUNG DISEASE

STEM: This baby has always had difficulty with breathing. Please examine his chest and tell us what you find.

PRESENTATION OF EXAMINATION FINDINGS

Duncan is a thin infant with reduced subcutaneous fat. He has scaphocephaly and a relatively high arched palate. There are multiple small scars on the dorsal aspects of both hands. He is in 0.2 litres of pernasal oxygen with saturations of 96%. He is pink with a respiratory rate of 40 breaths per minute and minimal nasal flaring. His chest is hyperinflated with mild intercostal and subcostal inspiratory recession. He has a left thoracotomy scar. There is good air entry with a combination of inspiratory crackles and expiratory wheeze. His liver edge is 2 cm below the costal margin. Duncan also has bilateral inguinal scars. I would like to plot his length, weight and head circumference on an appropriate centile chart using his corrected gestational age.

Thinking pause.....
In summary this is an ex-prem infant with evidence of chronic lung disease.

What is the benefit of antenatal corticosteroids?
The National Institutes of Health recommend the administration of antenatal corticosteroids to mothers of foetuses of 24–34 weeks' gestation who are at risk of preterm delivery. Ideally, it involves a course of two doses given 12 hours apart and at least more than 12 hours prior to delivery. The steroids stimulate foetal lung maturation and work by activating the fibroblasts, which in turn induce type II pneumocytes to release surfactant. They have been shown to reduce the mortality of premature infants due to RDS by 50%. Antenatal corticosteroids have also been shown to play a beneficial role in reducing the incidence of intraventricular haemorrhage.

What is the role of steroids in weaning from the ventilator?
Preterm infants may be ventilated for prolonged periods of time and eventually require to be weaned from the ventilator. Their response to weaning is influenced by disease severity, gestational age and caloric support, and requires careful monitoring. Various pharmacological agents are involved in the management of RDS to improve respiration – steroids and bronchodilators are the commonest. Static ventilator settings, minimal improvement in compliance, and increasing resistance are indicators for steroid therapy for infants 10 days or older who remain ventilated. Steroids are used for their anti-inflammatory effect in reducing oedema, white cell infiltration, fibroblast activation and the deposition of collagen. Latterly, there have been concerns that postnatal steroids are associated with increased risk of cerebral palsy. Although steroids reduce the amount of time the baby is ventilator dependent they do not affect the duration spent in hospital or the time the baby is oxygen dependent.

What do you think the left thoracotomy scar is from?
Preterm babies frequently have a significant persistent ductus arteriosus which fails to close spontaneously or with medical therapy (namely indometacin) and requires surgical ligation.

What are the important principles of management of an ex-preterm baby after discharge?
Optimal nutritional status is perhaps the most important area to ensure adequate growth. Feeds may even be supplemented with nasogastric feeds with supplements. Most babies will also receive vitamin and iron supplements. Normal childhood immunisations are particularly highlighted

and these children will also be eligible for pneumococcal vaccine and RSV monoclonal antibodies. It is important that the appropriate oxygen equipment is in place at home, with pulse oximetry for regular monitoring to keep the oxygen saturation greater than 95%, and the parents are comfortable with its use. Training of the parents in basic life support is mandatory. Emotional support for the parents is also essential. Regular follow-up of these babies, particularly for their developmental progress, is mandatory. Early recognition of intercurrent respiratory illness is important with a low threshold for admission to hospital.

FIBROSING ALVEOLITIS

STEM: This young boy is underweight and short of breath. Please examine his respiratory system and present your findings.

PRESENTATION OF EXAMINATION FINDINGS

Mark is a teenage boy who is thin with evidence of respiratory distress. He is mildly cyanosed, with finger clubbing and is tachypnoeic with a respiratory rate of 28 breaths per minute. He has a small scar at the right lung base posteriorly, most likely from a lung biopsy. His chest is symmetrical although expansion is reduced at the bases. There is no mediastinal shift. Percussion note is dull at both bases and he has fine inspiratory crackles at the lung bases bilaterally. He has a right parasternal heave and a loud pulmonary component to the second heart sound. There are no signs of Cushing's syndrome.

Thinking pause.....
Mark is a boy with fibrosing alveolitis and a degree of pulmonary hypertension.

Anything else?

These children generally fail to thrive. Thus I would like to assess his nutritional status and plot his height and weight on a growth chart appropriate for his age and sex. I would also like to assess his pubertal status as this is commonly delayed in these patients. I would also like a chest X-ray which, in the presence of fibrosing alveolitis, would demonstrate a diffuse ground glass appearance, and an ECG to look for evidence of right ventricular hypertrophy and right heart strain.

How would you manage this patient?

Most cases of fibrosing alveolitis are idiopathic, although occasionally it can be associated with connective tissue disorders. Treatment options are immunosuppression with corticosteroids, domiciliary oxygen if required, and optimising nutrition.

CHRONIC ASTHMA

STEM: This young boy with intermittent shortness of breath is under regular review by the respiratory paediatrician. Please examine his chest and tell us what you find.

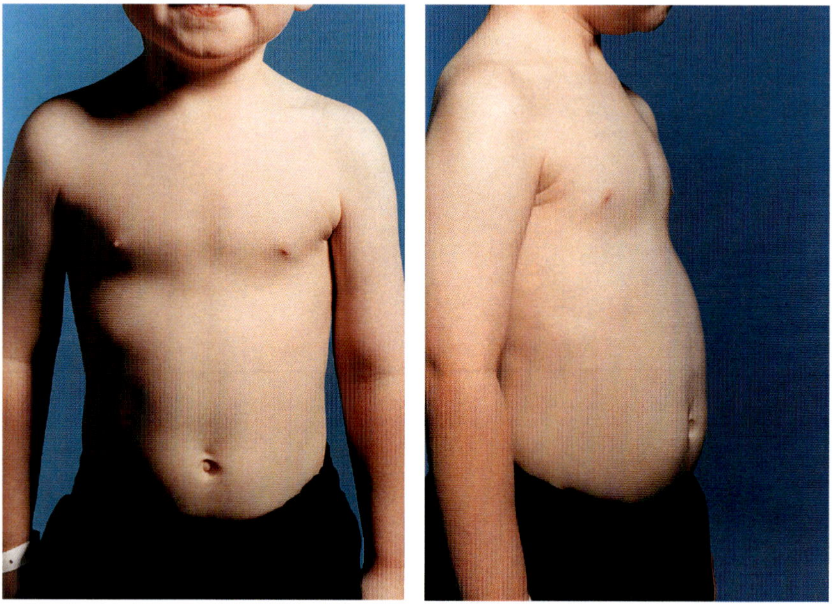

a b

Fig. 3.4 (**a, b**) *A boy with chronic asthma showing a hyperinflated chest with sternal depression and early development of a Harrison's sulcus.*

PRESENTATION OF EXAMINATION FINDINGS

Scott is a well-grown 6-year-old boy with no dysmorphic features. He is pink at rest in air and has no finger clubbing. He is undistressed with a respiratory rate of 20 breaths per minute. His chest is hyperinflated and he has a Harrison's sulcus and mild pectus carinatum. His trachea is central and his chest expansion symmetrical. Percussion note is resonant with vesicular breath sounds and no crackles or wheeze. He has a peak flow meter and a beta-agonist turbohaler by his bed.

Thinking pause.....
Scott is a young boy with chronic asthma who is currently well.

Anything else?
I would like to check his peak flow and compare it to his previous results. I would also like to plot his height and weight on a growth chart appropriate for his age and sex, as children with poorly controlled chronic asthma are

shorter than their peers. Atopy is also commonly encountered in these patients and Scott may have a history of eczema. It is also important to check his inhaler technique and ask his parents whether he also:

- has a device for prophylaxis?
- has required oral steroids over the last year and, if so, how frequently?
- has missed time from school?
- has coughing/waking during the night?
- has missed sports at school?

as well as how long his inhalers last him and whether they have a plan of management for an acute asthma attack.

4

THE GASTROINTESTINAL SYSTEM

ABDOMINAL EXAMINATION SUMMARY

INSPECTION
I would ideally like to expose the patient from nipples to knees

General
Dysmorphism, nutritional status, hair, jaundice, gastrostomy tubes, TPN lines, wearing nappies, scratch marks, spider naevi, bruising, race

Hands
Clubbing, pallor, xanthoma, leuconychia, koilonychia, palmar erythema

Face
Jaundice, pallor

Mouth
Pigmentation on lips, ulcers, dental caries, gum hypertrophy, macroglossia, cheilitis

Abdomen
- Distension (5 Fs): **f**at, **f**aeces, **f**luid, **f**latus, **f**oetus
- Scars: including renal, herniae, biopsy scars
- Visible organomegaly, caput medusa (veins drain away from umbilicus), distended abdominal veins
- Hernia including umbilical (commoner in Afro-Caribbean, Down's syndrome, MPS, hypothyroidism)
- Genitalia: hydrocele
- Nappy: stool colour, urine

PALPATION
Neck
Lymphadenopathy

Abdomen
Do not take your eyes off child's face
- Superficial and deep palpation in each of the quadrants.
- Hepatomegaly: size (use tape measure, not 'fingerbreadths'), smooth, tender, pulsatile (AV malformation), expansile (tricuspid regurgitation), splenomegaly, kidneys
- Know how to explain the difference between liver, spleen and kidneys

Percussion
Upper and lower borders of the liver, ascites

AUSCULTATION
Bowels sounds, renal bruits (hypertension, neurofibromatosis)

ANYTHING ELSE?
- Offer to examine the genitalia and also the anus for fistulae or skin tags
- Plot height and weight on a growth chart appropriate for age and sex
- Offer to inspect the stools and test the urine

Routine examination of the gastrointestinal system is straightforward but in the exam setting it has the potential to engender fear in the candidate because of ambiguity in the instruction. The examiner will give a brief history of the case and then ask the candidate to examine the child. When asked to examine or palpate the child's abdomen remember a few important points. In the older child, consider the patient's embarrassment when exposing the abdomen. Lowering the garments to just above the pubic symphysis is acceptable. When preparing the position of the patients use this time to perform your inspection of the patients and any visual clues around the bed. Although asked to examine the abdomen, it only takes a moment to examine the hands and face and probably quicker just to do so rather than ask the examiner if this is okay.

GASTROENTEROLOGY SHORT CASES

NUTRITIONAL ASSESSMENT

STEM: This 5-year-old boy is very underweight for his age. Please assess his nutritional status and present your findings.

PRESENTATION OF EXAMINATION FINDINGS

Dougal is a 5-year-old boy with a height of 108 cm, which lies on the 25th centile for his age and a weight of 10.5 kg, which lies below the 3rd centile for his age. He has reduced subcutaneous tissue and muscle wasting of his buttocks. He has generalised alopecia. His teeth and nails appear to be healthy. His mouth is clear with no ulcers or cheilitis. Dougal has an indwelling central venous access device and is receiving total parenteral nutrition. He is pale, with several bruises on his shins, arms and trunk but no other evidence to suggest chronic liver disease. His abdomen is soft and non-tender with no organomegaly, and bowel sounds are present. His bottom is excoriated.

Thinking pause.....
Dougal is a young boy who is malnourished and receiving total parenteral nutrition. In view of his alopecia and present nutritional status I would like to ask the parents if he is receiving chemotherapy treatment for cancer.

How would you assess nutritional status?
Assessment of nutritional status involves an evaluation of past and present dietary intake, anthropometry and laboratory assessments:

1. *Dietary assessment*: This would include details on the number of meals per day, including the typical meals and amounts taken. A more accurate

assessment can be obtained by asking the parents to keep a food diary for several days. From this an assessment of the calorie intake versus the expected calorie intake is made (kcal/kg/day), including a breakdown of protein, fat, carbohydrates, etc.

2. *Anthropometry*: Accurate assessment of nutrition is made by measuring the following:
   - Height – serial growth measurements are very helpful, as a fall in growth velocity is one of the earliest indicators of incipient malnutrition, but previous measurements are not always available.
   - Weight.
   - Triceps skin-fold thickness – this is an indicator of subcutaneous fat stores.
   - Mid-arm circumference – together with skin-fold thickness this is an indicator of skeletal muscle mass.
3. *Laboratory investigations*: This would involve measurement of electrolytes, vitamins and minerals, and immune status. Adaptation to malnutrition would be accompanied by low albumin and low levels of specific vitamins and minerals. Immunodeficiency, with low lymphocyte count and impaired cell-mediated immunity, is also associated with severe malnutrition. These findings are less important than history, examination and anthropometry.

When would you institute nutritional support?

Malnutrition is a common cause of death in developing countries and also occurs in developed countries as a consequence of poverty, poor education or parental neglect. In the hospital setting malnutrition is estimated to affect up to 40% of patients, and is particularly prevalent in chronically ill children with congenital heart disease, cystic fibrosis, inflammatory bowel disease, renal failure and cerebral palsy. In these conditions malnutrition is usually a consequence of anorexia, malabsorption and increased requirements secondary to infection or inflammation, and will usually respond to nasogastric tube feeding or by gastrostomy feeds. Total parenteral nutrition is often required for a period of time.

HEPATOMEGALY

STEM: This 5-year-old girl has been sent by her family doctor as she is short for her age and has feeding problems. Please examine her abdomen and tell us what you find.

PRESENTATION OF EXAMINATION FINDINGS

Pauline is a well-looking, 5-year-old girl with a rounded 'doll face', who appears small for her age. She has truncal obesity and muscle atrophy with a protuberant abdomen. The patient has bruises of different ages on her limbs. She also has a nasogastric tube in situ. There is no jaundice or pallor. Abdominal palpation revealed a smooth liver enlarging to below the umbilicus, measuring 12 cm. The kidneys are also moderately enlarged bilaterally. There is no associated splenomegaly or lymphadenopathy. I would like to plot Pauline's height and weight on a growth chart appropriate for her age and sex.

Thinking pause.....

Pauline's findings are in keeping with a diagnosis of glycogen storage disease. Given the picture of short stature, hepatomegaly and doll-face appearance the most likely underlying condition is von Gierke's disease or Type IA glycogen storage disorder.

Would you like to ask the parents a question?

'Does Pauline have a problem with low sugar levels in her body?'

How is this condition diagnosed?

GSDs are a group of recessively inherited disorders of carbohydrate metabolism. There are nine main enzyme defects which prevent the mobilisation of glucose from glycogen, either predominantly in muscle or in liver. In von Gierke's disease there is a deficiency of glucose-6-phosphatase preventing the dephosphorylation of glucose-6-phosphate into glucose. Provisional diagnosis can be made by demonstrating a fall in blood lactate from a high fasting level to near normal during an oral glucose tolerance test. Definitive diagnosis is made by biochemical assay of glucose-6-phosphatase activity in a needle liver biopsy. Antenatal diagnosis is not yet available. In this case the liver is the main organ affected due to a deficiency of glucose-6-phosphatase and hepatomegaly and hypoglycaemia are the characteristic features.

What are the important steps of management?

To prevent hypoglycaemia with a high carbohydrate diet, overnight nasogastric feeds, or in older children slow release oligosaccharides (corn starch). The parents must also be informed that the child will bruise easily and may have nose bleeds due to disordered platelet function. It is also important to ensure that this is Type IA as a similar condition (Type IB) involving a similar enzyme (glucose-6-phosphate translocase) results in metabolic abnormalities of leucocytes resulting in impaired phagocytosis, neutropenia and consequently an increased risk of severe infections – thus Type IB has a much poorer prognosis.

What complications are associated with the GSDs?

In Type I disease hyperuricaemia occurs due to shunting of the glucose-6-phosphate through the pentose–phosphate shunt to urate. Urate kidney stones and gout are prevented with the use of allopurinol but other renal problems occur, namely the more serious focal glomerulosclerosis.

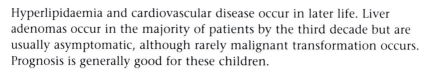

Hyperlipidaemia and cardiovascular disease occur in later life. Liver adenomas occur in the majority of patients by the third decade but are usually asymptomatic, although rarely malignant transformation occurs. Prognosis is generally good for these children.

Type II (Pompe) disease affects predominantly muscle and is associated with a poorer prognosis, with death from cardiomyopathy. The other types affect liver and muscle to a varying degree and have a good prognosis.

What are the causes of hepatomegaly?

This depends on the age of the child and the degree of hepatomegaly (Table 4.1).

Table 4.1 Causes of hepatomegaly

Cause	Type	Outcome
Infective	Congenital Acquired	CMV/toxoplasmosis, rubella Viral, e.g. CMV/EBV/hepatitis Protozoal, e.g. malaria
Haematological/ oncological	Benign Malignant	Haemolytic anaemias, e.g. HS Hepatoblastoma, haemangioendothelioma, leukaemia, lymphoma
Cardiac failure		
Storage disorders	CHO Amino acids Fat	MPS, GSD, galactosaemia Tyrosinaemia, urea cycle Gaucher's, Tay–Sach's, Niemann–Pick
Bile flow obstruction		Biliary atresia, gallstones
Autoimmune		CAH, UC, JIA, SLE
Drugs		Halothane, cytotoxic, valproate
Metabolic		α1-Antitrypsin deficiency, Wilson's, cystic fibrosis

SPLENOMEGALY

SICKLE CELL DISEASE

STEM: Do you think this young boy is jaundiced? Please examine him.

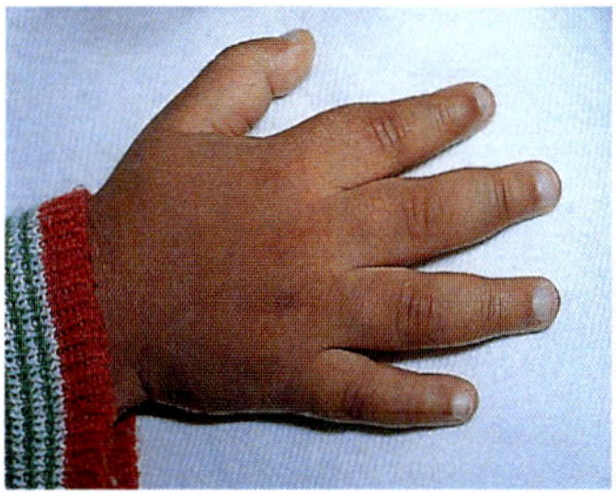

Fig. 4.1 *Swelling of the fingers from dactylitis (the hand–foot syndrome) is a common mode of presentation of sickle cell disease in late infancy.*
(Reproduced with kind permission from Lissauer T, Clayden G. Illustrated Textbook of Paediatrics, 2nd edn. Edinburgh: Mosby, 2001.)

PRESENTATION OF EXAMINATION FINDINGS

Osman is a young Afro-Caribbean boy with icteric sclerae and pale conjunctivae. He is comfortable at rest with no evidence of chronic liver disease. Abdominal examination revealed a 4 cm splenomegaly.

Thinking pause.....
The most likely diagnosis in this case is sickle cell disease.

What is the significance of this disease?
Sickle cell disease is one of the haemoglobinopathies, resulting from a single amino acid substitution (of valine for glutamine) at position 6 of the β chain, coded on chromosome 11. The condition is mainly found in people of African descent and is thought to offer protection against malaria. In the deoxygenated state the haemoglobin molecule becomes deformed and the red cell forms an irreversible sickle shape, which is trapped in the microcirculation and causes ischaemia. This is exacerbated by cold, dehydration and low oxygen concentration.

How may it present?
Sickle cell disease can manifest itself in one of several ways:

- *Anaemia*: There will usually be chronic moderate anaemia (Hb 6–8 g/dl) with jaundice due to chronic haemolytic haemolysis. This may also result in cardiomegaly.
- *Painful crisis*: This results from vascular occlusion and can affect any organ, with varying frequency and severity, although in young children vaso-occlusion often causes pain and swelling of the fingers and toes – dactylitis. Dactylitis is the presenting feature in 40% of patients and accounts for over 90% of acute admissions. Other common sites are femoral heads, limb and spinal bones. More serious, but fortunately less commonly, cerebral and pulmonary infarction or autosplenectomy can occur. In contrast to small vessel involvement in other parts of the body, cerebral infarction results from blockage of the medium to large arteries, and presents with acute hemiparesis.

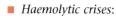

- *Haemolytic crises*:
  1. Aplastic crisis: precipitous drop in haemoglobin, usually secondary to parvovirus B19 (erythrovirus B19) infection causing marrow failure.
  2. Sequestration crisis: the sickle cells may accumulate in the spleen, resulting in rapid enlargement, pain and circulatory collapse, or in the lungs, resulting in circulatory failure.
- *Priapism*
- *Infection*: Autosplenectomy occurs during infancy, due to repeated subclinical splenic infarction, and significantly renders the child susceptible to infection from encapsulated organisms, particularly pneumococcus and *Haemophilus influenzae*. The risk of overwhelming sepsis is greatest in childhood. Osteomyelitis, particularly due to *Salmonella*, occurs more frequently in these children and there is also an increased risk of fulminant sepsis.

What are the long-term complications?

Pigmented gallstones from excessive bilirubin production are relatively common. The children are usually of short stature and may have pubertal delay. Cardiomegaly from chronic uncorrected anaemia may result in heart failure. Leg ulcers and renal impairment are also reported.

What are the mainstays of treatment?

1. *Prophylaxis*:
   - Warmth
   - Prevent dehydration
   - Penicillin prophylaxis is given from 3 months of age
   - Immunisations where appropriate:
     — pneumococcal polysaccharide and meningococcal a and c vaccinations are given from 2 years onwards. Pneumococcal conjugate vaccine if <2 years old.
     — standard *H. influenzae* type b, and meningococcal c conjugate vaccines are also given at 2, 3 and 4 months of age.
   - Daily folic acid is given to cope with the increased demands due to haemolysis
2. *Prompt treatment of acute crises*:
   - Warmth
   - Hydration
   - Oxygenation
   - Analgesia
   - Blood transfusions will abolish the pain and may also be required in haemolytic crises. This carries the standard risks of alloimmunisation (7–30%), transmission of infection and iron overload
   - Exchange transfusion, to reduce the proportion of sickle cells is indicated for neurological and pulmonary infarction and priapism
3. *Hydroxyurea*: This has been shown to reduce pulmonary crises and deaths by increasing HbF, red cell hydration, survival and deformability. It has also been shown to increase nitric oxide release and reduce endothelial red cell adhesion molecules (VCAM-1). It is not used routinely in the UK.
4. *Bone marrow transplant*: The current guidelines advocate BMT for patients under 16 years of age, with severe disease, who have an HLA-matched sibling.

5. *Nocturnal oxygen*: Studies have shown that patients are at increased risk of subclinical CNS damage, secondary to hypoxia, in the region of 20% by the age of 45 years. Based on the observation that 30% of children are hypoxic (sats <96%) overnight, new studies have been developed to look at the benefits of nocturnal oxygen.

What is the long-term outlook for these children?
The survival rate to the age of 20 years is in the region of 85%, the majority of deaths occurring in the first 3 years of life due to infection. BMT will provide a cure for these patients but the severity of their illness must be balanced against the side effects associated with BMT. Studies have shown disease-free survival rates in the region of 84%, with recurrence in approximately 10% of patients.

What is the advantage of antenatal or neonatal screening of at-risk groups?
This allows early administration of prophylaxis and parent education.

HEREDITARY SPHEROCYTOSIS

> **STEM:** This young girl's mother is concerned that she is pale. Please examine her abdomen and present your findings.

PRESENTATION OF EXAMINATION FINDINGS

Leigh is an 8-year-old girl with pallor and mild jaundice. She is otherwise well with no stigmata of chronic liver disease. Abdominal palpation revealed a 5 cm splenomegaly.

Thinking pause.....
The most likely diagnosis in this case is hereditary spherocytosis.

What is hereditary spherocytosis?
This is a haemolytic anaemia due to a disorder of the red cell membrane. It is an autosomal dominant disorder with variable penetrance. It presents with jaundice, generally in childhood, although it can present in the neonatal period. There is usually only mild anaemia except during intercurrent infections, particularly with parvovirus, which can lead to aplastic crisis. Pigmented gallstones due to increased bilirubin production also occur.

How is it managed?
As with other haemolytic anaemias, folic acid is required to cope with the increased demands. Blood transfusions may be required for the more serious aplastic crisis. If this is repeated excessively, splenectomy is an option.

What are the causes of splenomegaly?
This generally depends on the age and race of the patient and degree of splenomegaly but can usefully be classified as shown in Table 4.2.

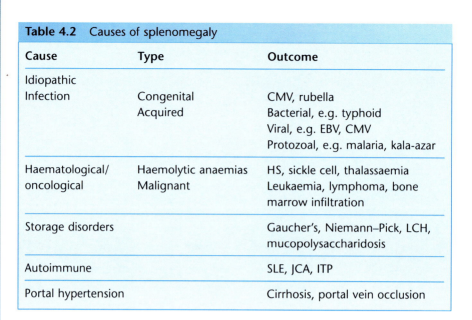

Table 4.2 Causes of splenomegaly

Cause	Type	Outcome
Idiopathic		
Infection	Congenital	CMV, rubella
	Acquired	Bacterial, e.g. typhoid
		Viral, e.g. EBV, CMV
		Protozoal, e.g. malaria, kala-azar
Haematological/ oncological	Haemolytic anaemias	HS, sickle cell, thalassaemia
	Malignant	Leukaemia, lymphoma, bone marrow infiltration
Storage disorders		Gaucher's, Niemann–Pick, LCH, mucopolysaccharidosis
Autoimmune		SLE, JCA, ITP
Portal hypertension		Cirrhosis, portal vein occlusion

HEPATOSPLENOMEGALY

STEM: This girl attends for regular blood transfusions. Please examine her abdomen and tell us what you find.

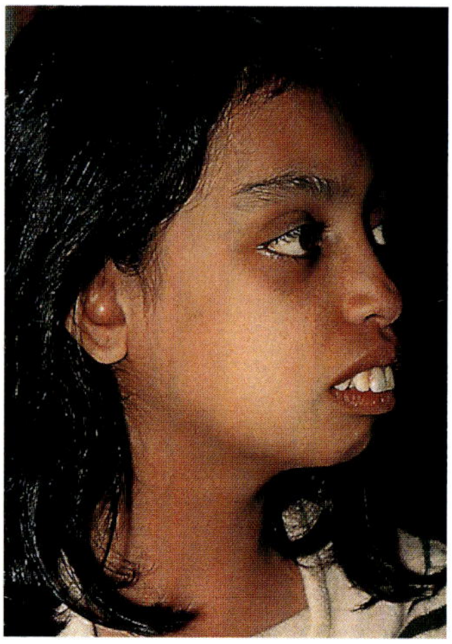

Fig. 4.2 *Facies in β-thalassaemia showing maxillary overgrowth and frontal skull bossing.*
(Reproduced with kind permission from Lissauer T, Clayden G. Illustrated Textbook of Paediatrics, 2nd edn. Edinburgh: Mosby, 2001.)

PRESENTATION OF EXAMINATION FINDINGS

Fatima is a 10-year-old girl with pallor and mild jaundice. She has frontal bossing and maxillary overgrowth. On her abdomen there are small scars. Abdominal palpation revealed marked hepatosplenomegaly with an 8 cm liver and a 10 cm spleen. I would also like to plot her height and weight on a growth chart appropriate for her age and sex, as I would anticipate that she is of short stature.

Thinking pause.....

These findings are in keeping with a diagnosis of β-thalassaemia major.

How is the diagnosis confirmed?

Haemoglobin electrophoresis will detect very high levels of HbF (90%), no HbA and increased or normal HbA2. Identifying carrier family members and genetic counselling is also essential.

How is it managed?

Chronic severe anaemia and jaundice are the norm from 6 months of age. Regular blood transfusions, every 3–4 weeks, are required once haemoglobin is <6 g/dl for 3 months to maintain haemoglobin concentration above 9–14 g/dl and suppress erythropoiesis, in order to reduce growth retardation, iron overloading, extramedullary haematopoiesis and bone deformation, resulting in the characteristic 'rodent faces'.

What are the complications of multiple blood transfusions?

As with all blood products, transfusion reactions can occur and thus leucocyte-depleted blood is used. Increased exposure increases the risk of antibody formation, either red cell or HLA antibodies. Repeated blood transfusions result in chronic iron deposition, as monitored by serum ferritin and consequently affects most systems. In particular, haemosiderosis leads to cardiomyopathy, liver cirrhosis, diabetes, hypoparathyroidism and skin hyperpigmentation. Prior to 1985 there was an increased risk of transmission of hepatitis C and HIV infection but blood is now screened for these infections in addition to hepatitis B. The issue of venous access can also pose a problem following repeated transfusions and sampling.

What are the scars on her abdomen from?

Repeated blood transfusion causes chronic iron overload. Daily overnight subcutaneous injections of the iron chelator desferrioxamine increase urinary excretion of iron and help to prevent haemosiderosis. However, desferrioxamine therapy predisposes to *Yersinia* infection. Daily vitamin C in small doses also helps to increase urinary iron excretion. For patients not complying with subcutaneous injections, oral iron chelation with deferiprone is possible but toxicity includes neutropenia, arthropathy and teratogenicity.

What are the options for treatment?

Generally, splenectomy is performed when signs of hypersplenism appear as indicated by the need for transfusions in excess of 240 ml/kg of packed cells per year. Bone marrow transplantation is an option for those children who have an HLA-compatible sibling donor. BMT results in cure for these patients but it is not without significant mortality and morbidity. Delayed puberty occurs in 50% of patients and conditioning with gonadotoxic chemotherapy causes infertility in the majority of patients.

CIRRHOSIS AND PORTAL HYPERTENSION

STEM: This young boy has had a lot of abdominal surgery and hospitalisation in his short life. Please examine him and tell us what you find.

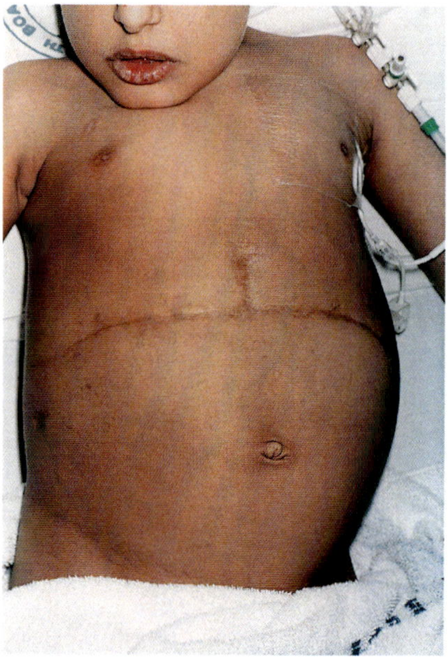

Fig. 4.3 *This boy is jaundiced with a grossly distended abdomen and dilated abdominal veins. He has an old transverse, hypochondrial scar ('roof-top incision') and a previous liver biopsy scar. He has an indwelling central venous access device (Hickman line).*

PRESENTATION OF EXAMINATION FINDINGS

Ewan is a thin, 7-year-old boy with loss of muscle bulk. He is jaundiced with scratch marks on his forearms. He has a grossly distended abdomen with dilated abdominal veins. Abdominal palpation revealed a 4 cm splenomegaly with no hepatomegaly. He has abdominal ascites as confirmed by shifting dullness. There is a transverse, hypochondrial old scar.

Thinking pause.....
This is a young boy with portal hypertension and evidence of major abdominal surgery.

What is the scar from?

This boy may have undergone a liver transplant for biliary atresia. Biliary atresia is characterised by obstructive jaundice secondary to destruction or absence of the extrahepatic bile ducts. If untreated it progresses to involve the intrahepatic biliary tree leading to chronic liver failure and death. Surgical treatment involves a hepatoportal enterostomy (Kasai procedure) to bypass the obliterated ducts and allow free bile drainage. This is achieved in 80% if the operation is performed within the first 60 days of life. In those patients in whom this is unsuccessful or only temporarily successful liver transplantation is necessary.

What is the cause of ascites?

The pathogenesis of ascites is incompletely understood and is thought to be a combination of hypoalbuminaemia, sodium retention and impaired renal function. Salt and fluid intake is restricted and diuretics are used to control mild ascites. Albumin infusions with diuretics can be used to expand the intravascular volume and, very rarely, paracentesis may be required if there is gross abdominal distension compromising ventilation. Peritoneovenous shunts may be used for refractory ascites.

How would you manage chronic liver disease?

The mainstay of treatment is supportive in terms of ensuring adequate nutrition and preventing complications. Anorexia is a common problem but it is essential to provide a high-protein, high-carbohydrate diet with adequate essential fatty acids, vitamins and minerals. Up to a 50% increase in calories above the standard for weight is often required to prevent malnutrition and feeding may be supplemented with nasogastric or parenteral feeds. Pruritus is a common symptom and the patient is afforded some relief with colestyramine. Spontaneous bacterial peritonitis and encephalopathy are two important complications which require early diagnosis and intervention.

What are the indications for liver transplantation?

Liver transplantation is a therapeutic option in chronic end-stage liver failure, which is unresponsive to intensive nutritional supplementation resulting in severe malnutrition and inadequate growth, or associated with a poor quality of life. Studies have shown an overall 1-year survival of 90% with a 5-year survival of 75%. Liver transplantation requires lifelong immunosuppression with long-term follow-up.

WILSON'S DISEASE

STEM: This 9-year-old boy has been failing to thrive and complaining of abdominal pain. His teachers also report that he is beginning to fall behind with his classwork. Please examine his GI system and tell us what you find.

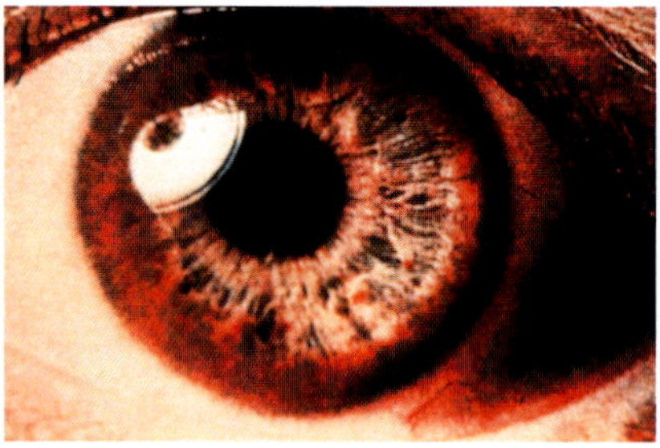

Fig. 4.4 *Kayser–Fleischer rings from copper in the cornea of a child with Wilson's disease.*
(Reproduced with kind permission from Lissauer T, Clayden G. Illustrated Textbook of Paediatrics, 2nd edn. Edinburgh: Mosby, 2001.)

PRESENTATION OF EXAMINATION FINDINGS

Tim is a malnourished 9-year-old boy with reduced subcutaneous fat and loss of muscle bulk. He has palmar and plantar erythema and spider naevi. His tone is generally reduced. The most striking feature is abdominal distension and scrotal swelling and on palpation there is splenomegaly. Percussion and shifting dullness confirm ascites.

Thinking pause.....
This is a boy with chronic liver disease and portal hypertension.

Anything else?
I would like to plot his height and weight on a growth chart appropriate for his age and sex. I would also like to perform slit lamp examination of his eyes to exclude Kayser–Fleischer rings on the cornea as a possible underlying diagnosis may be Wilson's disease.

What is Wilson's disease?
This is an autosomal recessive disorder with the defective gene on chromosome 13 with an incidence of 1 in 200 000 births. This inborn error of metabolism is characterised by a combination of reduced synthesis of the copper binding protein caeruloplasmin, and defective biliary excretion of copper with consequent accumulation of copper in the liver, brain, cornea and kidney. The clinical presentation of liver disease varies from acute hepatitis to the insidious development of cirrhosis and portal hypertension. Often children present with altered behaviour and deteriorating school performance, and extrapyramidal signs are present from the second decade. Other diagnostic pointers include haemolytic anaemia and renal tubular dysfunction, with vitamin D resistant rickets.

How is the diagnosis confirmed?
Confirmation is the finding of low caeruloplasmin, low serum copper, excess urinary copper excretion with a further increase following a penicillamine load. Liver biopsy confirms increased accumulation of copper.

What is the treatment?

Penicillamine in combination with zinc reduces copper absorption. Pyridoxine is also given to prevent peripheral neuropathy. A low copper diet is also important. Up to 50% of children presenting in childhood have liver disease so advanced that liver transplantation is the treatment of choice. Screening of siblings is essential once the index case is identified in order that early treatment can be started.

INFLAMMATORY BOWEL DISEASE

STEM: Claire was referred by her family doctor with a history of weight loss, recurrent abdominal pain and bloody diarrhoea. Please examine her abdomen and tell us what you find.

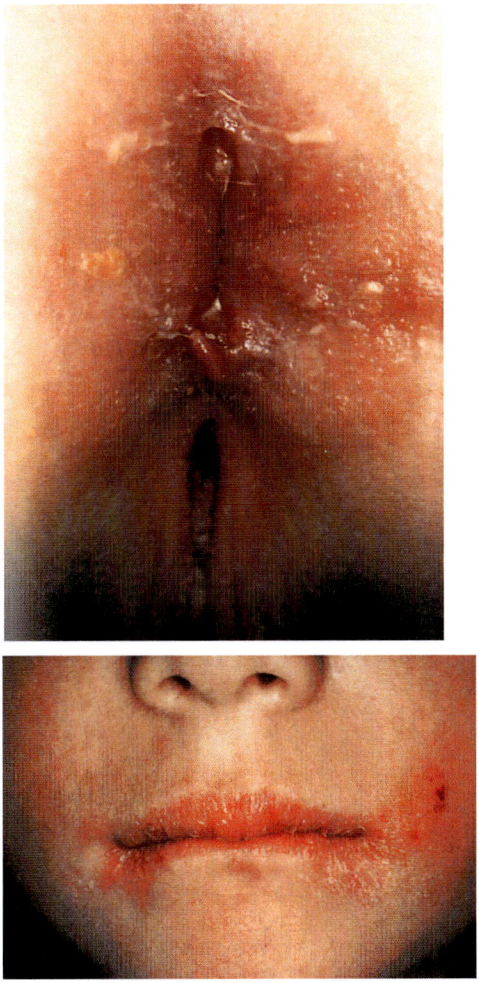

a

b

Fig. 4.5 *Inflammatory bowel disease.* (**a**) *Perineal inflammation and fistula;* (**b**) *stomatitis.* (Reproduced with kind permission from Milner D, Herber S. Self Assessment in Paediatrics. Edinburgh: Mosby, 1997.)

PRESENTATION OF EXAMINATION FINDINGS

Claire is a small, thin, pale 9-year-old girl with swelling of her lips and angular stomatitis. Claire has small aphthous ulcers on her buccal mucosa. She has a central venous long-line in situ. Claire has erythema nodosum on the anterior aspects of her lower legs. The lesions are erythematous, tender nodules of varying size and are hot to touch. She has no joint pain or swelling and no stigmata of liver disease. Examination of her abdomen was normal. She has no evidence of long-term steroid use. I would like to examine her anus for perianal skin tags, fissures, fistulae and abscesses and to plot her height and weight on a growth chart appropriate for her age and sex.

Thinking pause.....

Claire is a 9-year-old girl with some of the characteristic features of inflammatory bowel disease; in view of the mouth involvement, the most likely diagnosis is Crohn's disease.

How might you investigate a patient with suspected inflammatory bowel disease?

This would involve a combination of haematological, biochemical and radiological investigations in the first instance, followed by upper and lower endoscopy and biopsies.

1. *Haematology/clinical chemistry*:
   - FBC and film (MCV):
     - — iron deficiency anaemia is common
     - — white cell count may be raised and neutrophils elevated
     - — thrombocytosis is commonly found.
   - Acute phase reactants: ESR and CRP.
   - Liver function tests may be deranged: hypoalbuminaemia is common.
   - Ferritin, folate, vitamin B12, vitamins A, D, E, K, calcium, phosphate, copper, magnesium and zinc may be helpful in monitoring IBD.

   In acute colitis, prolonged diarrhoea may cause dehydration, hypokalaemia and acidosis.
2. *Radiological investigations*:
   - Plain abdominal X-ray – in acute situation:
     - — to exclude toxic megacolon suspected
     - — may reveal evidence of obstruction or dilatation, thickening of bowel wall or stones.
   - Abdominal ultrasound scan: small and large bowel wall thickening, nodal enlargement, abscesses, stones, fistulae.
   - Barium meal and follow through in Crohn's bowel involvement:
     - — patchy with cobblestone-like pattern of thickened small bowel wall
     - — fistula formation
     - — skip lesions, lumen narrowing, thickening and fissuring ('rose-thorn ulcers') are typical of Crohn's (but may be seen in chronic granulomatous disease).
   - Barium enema: in ulcerative colitis a barium enema usually shows a diffuse continuous distal lesion confined to the rectum and colon. Not the investigation of choice.

- White cell scans: not a first line investigation.
- Endoscopy procedures: as part of the diagnostic workup upper endoscopy may help diagnose CD from UC with the presence of characteristic histological changes on biopsy of the upper GI tract.

Once a diagnosis of Crohn's disease is made for Claire, what is the mainstay of her management?

IBD is a chronic condition that requires treatment by a multidisciplinary team including the gastroenterologist, nurse, dietician, social worker, psychologist, pharmacist, biochemist, microbiologist. This depends to a large extent on patient cooperation. Patients and their families require education about the illness and a great deal of support. The aim of treatment is to induce and maintain remission.

In the acute illness nutritional support and steroids are the mainstay of treatment. Aggressive enteral nutritional therapy is effective in inducing remission in Crohn's disease (usually small bowel disease patients) in up to 70–80% of cases. Steroids can induce remission in >80% of Crohn's disease. This is generally intravenous hydrocortisone 1 mg/kg four times daily or oral prednisolone 1 mg/kg/day, up to maximum 60 mg per day (most children maximum 40 mg), gradually tapered after remission gained and usually tapered after 4 weeks. Topical steroids – liquid or more usually foam enemas – can be used for disease confined to the left side of the colon, sigmoid colon and rectum.

Broad spectrum antibiotics (cefotaxime and metronidazole, or ampicillin, gentamicin and metronidazole) may be used when a colitic presents acutely, as there may be abscess or bacterial translocation in inflamed gut, but the majority use no antibiotics unless there are specific worries (many IBD patients are febrile but are culture negative). Metronidazole is effective in terminal ileal and particularly perianal disease, although peripheral neuropathy may develop with long-term use. Often, ciprofloxacin is used in addition to metronidazole, usually in a 2- to 3-month course.

What are the options if the patient fails to respond to steroids?

Immunomodulators are used for patients who either do not respond to steroids or those who respond but seem to be dependent on steroids (those who flare on tapering), and have been shown to have benefit in both Crohn's and UC.

- Azathioprine (usually next used after steroids, dose up to 2 mg/kg/day); some use 6-mercaptopurine, of which azathioprine is a prodrug. Generally used for a minimum of 4 years when started.
- Ciclosporin/tacrolimus may be used as a 'rescue' drug intravenously in acute colitis, with 50% gaining remission, but many tend to relapse after discontinuation. It has been associated with increased BP, hypomagnesaemia, seizures. Needs drug level monitoring, PCP prophylaxis.
- Methotrexate (used after azathioprine if no response, either oral, or usually subcutaneously once weekly).

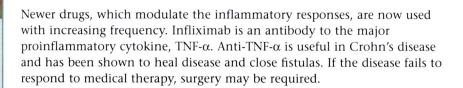

Newer drugs, which modulate the inflammatory responses, are now used with increasing frequency. Infliximab is an antibody to the major proinflammatory cytokine, TNF-α. Anti-TNF-α is useful in Crohn's disease and has been shown to heal disease and close fistulas. If the disease fails to respond to medical therapy, surgery may be required.

What measures can we take to maintain remission?

While steroids are very effective in the acute situation there is no evidence to suggest that low dose steroid therapy can maintain remission in Crohn's disease. Aminosalicylate (ASA) preparations have shown marginal long-term benefit for remission maintenance in Crohn's disease.

What is the long-term prognosis for this condition?

Most IBD patients suffer relapsing episodes of varying severity: some have mild disease and are seldom troubled, whereas some have very debilitating disease requiring multiple surgery, sometimes ending with short gut syndrome and lifelong parenteral nutrition dependence. Crohn's is associated with an increased risk of cancer but regular colonoscopic surveillance as in UC is not yet advocated.

You observed that Claire was of short stature. What is the effect of IBD on growth?

In one recent study, growth was impaired in >50% of cases, with approximately 25% of cases falling in the category of short stature. However, endocrine function tests demonstrate normal growth hormone secretion. The typical pattern is of growth retardation associated with delayed skeletal maturation. Cytokines have a deleterious effect on the cartilage growth plate and patients have been shown to have reduced levels of IGF-1. Puberty is also delayed in a significant number.

JAUNDICE

STEM: This infant was referred by his family doctor for further assessment of prolonged jaundice. Please examine him and tell us what you find.

PRESENTATION OF EXAMINATION FINDINGS

Richard is a 3-month-old infant with a prominent forehead, deep-set eyes with upward-sloping palpebral fissures. He has a prominent nasal bridge and a pointed chin. He is jaundiced with evidence of pruritus and he has pale stools in his nappy. On examination of his abdomen he has a small, relatively fresh scar in his right hypochondrial area and he has an 8 cm hepatomegaly. Cardiac auscultation reveals a 3/6 ESM over the pulmonary area.

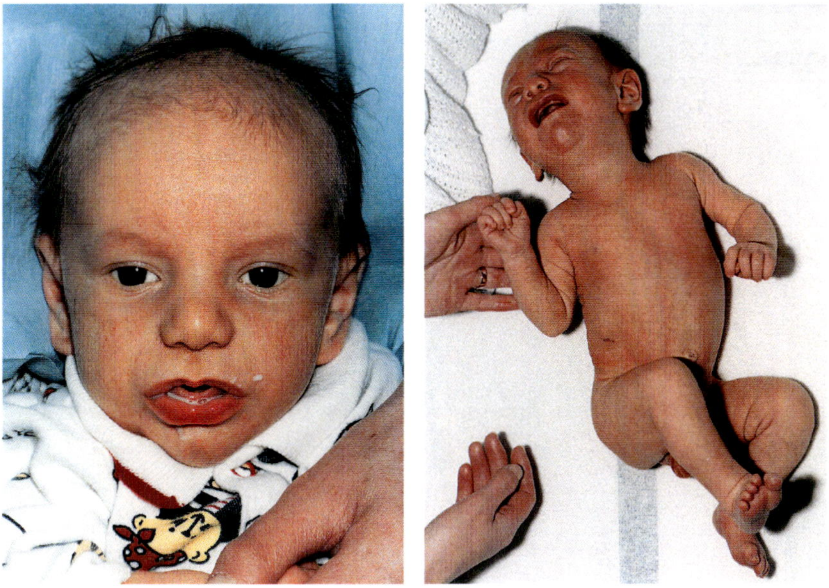

a b

Fig. 4.6 (**a**, **b**) *A baby with jaundice and icteric sclerae.* (**a**) *Note the facial features characteristic of Alagille syndrome – prominent forehead, deep-set eyes, mildly upward-sloping palpebral fissures, a prominent nasal bridge and a pointed chin.*

Thinking pause.....

This is a baby with jaundice, which is clinically most likely to be obstructive, a murmur in keeping with pulmonary stenosis and characteristic facial appearance in keeping with a diagnosis of Alagille syndrome. I would also like to ask if he has had an ophthalmology assessment of his eyes for posterior embryotoxin in the lens. He appears to have already undergone a liver biopsy.

How would you confirm your diagnosis of Alagille syndrome in Richard?

Defining the extent of the absence of extrahepatic ducts is done by isotope scanning of the liver (IDA scan: technetium 99m iminodiacetic acid) which will demonstrate uptake of the isotope by the liver but no excretion into the bowel at 24 hours. Liver biopsy will also demonstrate the paucity of bile ducts. Diagnosis of Alagille syndrome is by chromosomal analysis. Alagille syndrome is an autosomal dominant condition resulting from mutations in the JAG1 gene on chromosome 20p12 (2;3). JAG1 codes for a NOTCH receptor ligand which is important in cell–cell interactions and development.

What is Alagille syndrome?

This is a syndrome of intrahepatic bile duct hypoplasia leading to obstructive jaundice. Cardiac lesions are commonly associated with Alagille syndrome and are usually pulmonary stenosis or tetralogy of Fallot. These children often require liver transplantation (see previous case, Cirrhosis and portal hypertension, p. 50).

5
THE NERVOUS SYSTEM

It is with some trepidation that candidates approach the neurological examination in children. When examining the nervous system it is easier to think of it as a series of examinations which depend upon the age and ability of the child and the specific request of the examiner. The major categories are as follows:

- Examination of the cranial nerves
- Neurological examination of a baby/toddler
- Neurological examination of an older child
- Neurological examination of limb girdle and trunk (older child)
- Examination of the cerebellar system
- Examination of the child in a wheelchair.

EXAMINATION OF THE CRANIAL NERVES

Generally you will not be asked to examine all the cranial nerves in the exam but you may be asked to examine any of the individual nerves or components

CRANIAL NERVE I
Not directly tested; ask older child if any problems smelling food

CRANIAL NERVE II
Visual acuity Need to know if they can see and understand instructions. Begin with Snellen chart or print (for older child) and work down via counting fingers, detecting hand movement, distinguishing light from dark. The candidate who completely fails to realise a child is blind in one eye and progresses through a complex exam is not uncommon
Pupils Direct and consensual
Visual fields Confrontation perimetry in older child, each eye in turn; younger child may need two examiners – one to distract and the other to bring toy into child's periphery from behind
Fundoscopy Do this at the end

CRANIAL NERVES III, IV and VI
Eye movements 'Follow my finger with your eyes, keeping your head still. Tell me if you can see two fingers at any point.'

CRANIAL NERVE V
Motor 'Open your mouth – don't let me close it.' Feel masseters with teeth clenched (increased in Duchenne muscular dystrophy)
Sensory Test light touch in each of the three divisions: 'Close your eyes, say "yes" when you feel me touch you. Is it the same on both sides?'

CRANIAL NERVE VII
Motor 'Raise your eyebrows, screw your eyes up tight as if there is soap in them.' 'Puff out your cheeks.' 'Give me a big smile and show me your teeth.' Corneal reflex not tested as too painful
Sensory Supplies taste to anterior two-thirds of the tongue, seldom tested

CRANIAL NERVE VIII

Cochlear Examine external auditory meati for local disease, wax, grommets. Normal speech? In young infant lying down you can clap or ring bell and see if turns head to sound; in sitting child use distraction hearing test

- *Weber's test* – 512 Hz tuning fork in centre of frontal bone:
  — perceptive deafness: louder on healthy side
  — conductive deafness: louder on diseased side
- *Rinne's test* – 512 Hz tuning fork placed on mastoid bone:
  — conductive deafness: bone is louder
  — perceptive deafness or normal hearing: air louder

Vestibular Nystagmus can be checked for when assessing eye movements

CRANIAL NERVES IX and X

'Gag reflex' – generally not tested but ask patient to say 'ah' and observe for symmetrical elevation of the palatal arches. Voice dysphonia. Swallowing intact. Sensation to posterior third of tongue, soft palate, nasopharynx (IX) not tested for

CRANIAL NERVE XI

- 'Can you shrug your shoulders?' Any muscle wasting?
- 'Turn your head against my hand to look over your shoulder.'

CRANIAL NERVE XII

'Can you stick out your tongue?'

NEUROLOGICAL EXAMINATION OF A BABY/TODDLER

INSPECTION (Fully dressed on parent's lap)

1. Overall size and proportions head/trunk/limbs
2. Dysmorphic features
3. Posture – asymmetrical – alarm bells
4. Movement – gross and fine movement, sitting/standing:
   — general paucity
   — asymmetrical
   — accessory: tic, chorea, tremor, titubation, athetoid
   — convulsive

EYES

Start here as the child may cry

1. Eye-to-eye contact
2. Fixate?
3. Conjugate or squint?
4. Nystagmus/ptosis/cataract/iris/conjunctiva, etc.
5. Pupils

6. Test external ocular movements with toy (fix and follow 180° by 4 months)

OTHER CRANIAL NERVES

- VII – observe symmetry of smile
- VII, IX, X, XII – suck and swallow
- VII, X, XII – speech:
  — stammers relatively common and unrelated to pathology
  — delayed: learning difficulties, autism
  — difficult to understand (dysarthria much commoner than dysphasia): cerebral palsy, speech disorder
  — monotonous: deafness
- XII – stick out tongue

HEAD

1. Shape
2. Sutures
3. Fontanelles
4. Size – measure OFC at end
5. Feel for VP shunt/reservoir

HANDS

1. Dysmorphic – syndactyly, polydactyly, clinodactyly, palmar creases
2. Muscle wasting
3. Handedness (1½–5 yrs) if <18 months think hemiplegia
4. Offer child a toy – does he reach/grasp, is there any tremor, does he transfer?

NOW UNDRESS TO NAPPY (If >3 yrs in nappy ask why)

Simultaneously look for: muscle wasting, scars for VP shunts, scoliosis, lower spine abnormalities

ARMS

INSPECTION

1. Deformity (bony and soft tissue, skin markings)
2. Muscle bulk
3. Posture

TONE

- Increased = spasticity = UMNL = cerebral palsy in exams
- Decreased/absent = LMNL/neuromuscular junction, muscle disorder

POWER

- Tightness of grasping object
- Pull infant up by arms to supine

COORDINATION

Observe play, particularly watching the child's gait, manipulation of toys and ability to reach for toys successfully

REFLEXES
Increased in UMNL ± clonus; absent in LMNL

SENSATION
Not done in exams unless indicated or specifically asked for

TRUNK
- Sit from supine and observe balance
- Skin – abnormal skin markings suggesting TS of NF
- Sacrum/spine

LEGS
- **Always** start with gait – look for limp, broad based, spastic, hemiplegic (circumduction and foot scuffs the floor), waddling, toe-walking
- As for arms – inspection, tone, power, coordination and reflexes

NEUROLOGICAL EXAMINATION OF AN OLDER CHILD

INSPECTION (As for infant)
1. Overall size and proportions head/trunk/limbs
2. Dysmorphic features
3. Posture – asymmetrical – may indicate underlying pathology
4. Movement – gross and fine movement, sitting/standing:
   - — general paucity
   - — asymmetrical
   - — accessory: tic, chorea, tremor, titubation, athetoid
   - — convulsive

ARMS (Undress to the waist)

INSPECTION
- 'Hold your arms out straight like this.' Look for wasting, fasciculation, involuntary movements
- 'Which hand do you write with?'
- 'Stretch out your arms and play the piano like this.' Look for asymmetry

Always examine the normal side first.

TONE
Ask if it would hurt to move the arm

POWER
- Ask the child to bend his arms and hold them up at 90° out to the side:
  C5 (shoulder abduction) 'Push your elbows away from your body.'
  C6–8 (shoulder adduction) 'Pull your elbows into your body.'
- Bend arms so that elbow is at right angle:
  C5,6 (elbow flexion) 'Pull me towards you.'
  C7,8 (elbow extension) 'Push me away.'

- Ask the child to make a fist:
  C6,7 (wrist flexion/extension) 'Don't let me bend your wrist.'
- Ask the child to spread his fingers:
  T1 (finger abduction) 'Don't let me squeeze them together.'

COORDINATION

- Finger to nose touching
- Dysdiadochokinesis – show the child that you want him/her to tap one hand with the other, alternatively tapping the palm and the back of the hand

REFLEXES

Use the Jendrassik manoeuvre if it is difficult to elicit the reflexes and there are no other abnormal signs. Demonstrate to the child that you want him/her to screw up his/her face (or to pull his/her hands against each other if testing leg reflexes) on your command, just before you strike the tendon

SENSATION (Not done unless requested)

Light touch, proprioception

LEGS (Expose from groin downwards)

INSPECTION

Also have a quick look at the child's face for any clues such as myopathy or drooling. Look for muscle wasting, asymmetry, limp, fasciculation, foot drop, deformity

GAIT

- By 3 yrs: able to – walk on heels/tip-toes, run, stand on one leg for 5 seconds
- By 4 yrs: able to hop
- By 5 yrs: able to walk in a straight line for 20 steps
- By 7 yrs:
  - — tandem walking (heel–toe walking)
  - — Fog test: child walks on lateral borders of feet and hands also noted to turn inwards – suggestive of cerebral lesion
  - — 'crouch down' (distal muscles); 'now stand' (proximal muscles)

TONE

Increased = spasticity = cerebral palsy

POWER

'I'm going to test how strong you are':

L1,2: 'Lift your leg off the bed, keep it there and don't let me push it down.'
L5,S1: 'Push your leg into the bed, don't let me lift it off the bed.'
L3,4: 'Bend your knee, now try to straighten your leg out as if you are kicking me.'
S1: 'Bend your knee and try to pull your heel up towards your bottom.'
L4,5: 'Pull your toes up towards your head.'
L5: 'Pull your big toe up towards your head.'
S1,2: 'Point your toes towards the bed.'
L4,5: 'Turn your foot inwards.'
L5,S1: 'Turn your foot outwards.'

COORDINATION
Heel–shin test

REFLEXES
Remember reinforcement with the Jendrassik manoeuvre

SENSATION
Light touch:
L1: Inguinal ligament
L2: Middle of anterior thigh
L3: Medial aspect of knee
L4: Medial calf
L5: Lateral calf
S1: Sole of foot
S3–5: Perineal sensation (don't test unless you suspect an abnormality)

ANYTHING ELSE?
Spine, head (posterior fossa scar), joints

NEUROLOGICAL EXAMINATION OF LIMB GIRDLE AND TRUNK (OLDER CHILD)

SHOULDER GIRDLE
'Show me how you would comb your hair.'

TRUNK
'Can you lie on your back and sit up without using your hands?'

PELVIC GIRDLE
'Kneel down on the floor, now stand up without using your hands.'

GOWER'S SIGN
'Lie on your back, now try to stand up without using your hands.' Child rolls onto his front and then pushes up against his legs to get up, i.e. 'climbing up his legs'

EXAMINATION OF THE CEREBELLAR SYSTEM

DYSARTHRIA
'Hello, what's your name?' Chat to patient to assess speech

NYSTAGMUS
'Look straight ahead at me.' Are the eyes steady?
'Follow my finger with your eyes, keeping your head still.'

DYSDIADOCHOKINESIS
Show the child that you want him/her to tap one hand with the other, alternatively tapping the palm and the back of the hand

DYSMETRIA
The child will overshoot the target when asked to point to a target

INTENTION TREMOR
'Reach out and touch my finger.' The child's hand is steady at rest but develops a tremor of increasing amplitude as it approaches its target

ATAXIC GAIT
Ask the child to walk to the end of the ward and back. Look for broad-based gait with arms stretched out sideways for balance; difficulty turning corners

ROMBERG'S SIGN
'Stand with your feet together, close your eyes.' Positive if child become unsteady, due to loss of proprioception (rare in children)

EXAMINATION OF THE CHILD IN A WHEELCHAIR

INSPECTION
- Overall posture, use of wedges for support (hypotonia)
- Head size, hydrocephalus ± shunt (spina bifida)
- Face – dysmorphic features, myopathy
- Shake hands – feel for tone, grip, power and release of grip
- Urinary catheter bag (spina bifida)
- Splints, supports, callipers (cerebral palsy)

PALPATE
Feel scalp for a shunt/reservoir

DO NOT EXAMINE IN THE WHEELCHAIR
Explain to the examiner you would like to examine the patient on the bed – he may ask you to examine the upper limbs and arms only

TRY TO DETERMINE THE SITE OF PARESIS
- Head
- Cord
- Peripheral nerve
- Muscular disease

BELL'S PALSY

STEM: This girl's parents are concerned that she may have had a stroke. Can you examine her and tell us what you find?

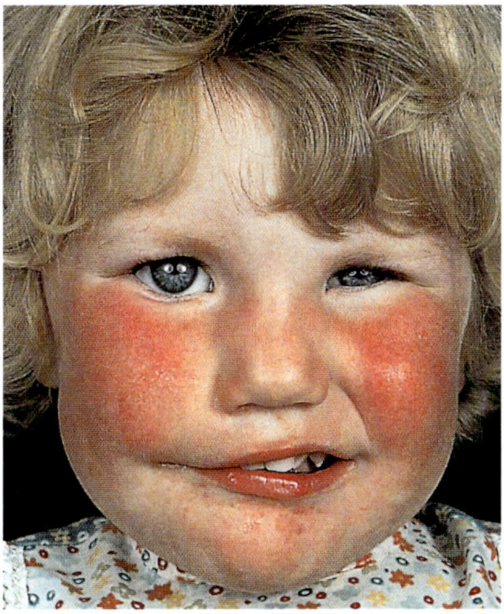

Fig. 5.1 *Bell's palsy. There is right facial weakness of both the upper and lower face.* (Reproduced with kind permission from Lissauer T, Clayden G. Illustrated Textbook of Paediatrics, 2nd edn. Edinburgh: Mosby, 2001.)

PRESENTATION OF EXAMINATION FINDINGS

Catrina is a 7-year-old girl with weakness of the muscles of the whole of the right side of her face. Her right eyelid does not close (Bell's phenomenon), the nasolabial crease is lost and the right side of her face does not move with voluntary, reflex or emotional movements. Facial sensation is normal. There is no local facial tenderness. This is in keeping with a right lower motor VIIth nerve palsy. The remainder of the cranial nerves are intact.

Thinking pause.....
This is a girl with Bell's palsy.

Anything else?
I would like to ask the parents if Catrina has a history of a recent viral infection. I would also like to test for taste sensation on the anterior two-thirds of her tongue and to measure her blood pressure. I would like to examine her auditory canals for the presence of herpes simplex vesicles.

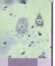

How would you treat acute onset of this condition?

In the acute phase it is important to control the pain and prevent corneal infection, abrasion or drying of the eye. In chronic cases of facial palsy, chloramphenicol eye drops, sellotaping of the eye and artificial tears may be necessary. In acute Bell's palsy steroids may be used but leukaemia, hypertension, brainstem tumours and middle ear disease must be excluded first. The rationales for using steroids are the anti-inflammatory effect to reduce oedema around the facial nerve and the immunosuppressant effect. Steroids must be given early in large doses to have any effect but only a few cases actually present within the first 48 hours. If there is a possibility that the condition may be due to herpes simplex virus infection (Ramsay Hunt syndrome), then aciclovir is given in addition to steroids, as steroids on their own would exacerbate the HSV infection. However, two-thirds will resolve spontaneously without treatment over the next 3 weeks. Progress can occur over the next few months but a few patients are left with mild facial asymmetry.

MACROCEPHALY

STEM: Christopher's parents have always been concerned that his head is too big. Please examine him.

PRESENTATION OF EXAMINATION FINDINGS

Christopher is a well-nourished toddler with no obvious dysmorphic features. His head size appears to be disproportionately large compared to his height, although I would like to measure his head circumference, height and weight and plot his measurements on a centile chart appropriate for his age and sex. I would also like to plot his parents' head circumferences. On palpation of his scalp he has a reservoir in situ and a shunt, which appears to be a ventriculoperitoneal shunt as he has a small scar in the right upper quadrant of his abdomen. His sutures are closed and his head shape is symmetrical although it is large. He has no distended scalp veins or sunsetting eyes, suggesting that there is no increased intracranial pressure at present. For a toddler, he is chatting away appropriately and his parents have no concerns about his hearing. He can walk and run and is able to pick up small objects with a neat pincer grip. He enjoys looking at pictures in the book and is interested in playing with bricks.

Thinking pause.....

This is a young boy with shunted hydrocephalus who does not have any dysmorphic features and appears to be developing appropriately. I would like to ask his parents if he was born prematurely and if there is any history of an intracranial bleed during that time, or any history of infection.

How you would classify macrocephaly?

I would divide the causes of a large head into normotensive and hypertensive as shown in Table 5.1.

What is the most likely cause of hydrocephaly in this child?

If Christopher was born at full term with a normal neonatal period, and given his apparently normal development and lack of other neurological

Table 5.1 Classification of macrocephaly

Classification	Category	Association
Normotensive		
Large brain (megalencephaly)	Anatomical	Normal variant – large baby Familial Associated with dwarfism – achondroplasia Associated with gigantism – Soto's syndrome (often developmentally delayed)
	Metabolic	Storage diseases, e.g. maple syrup urine disease, mucopolysaccharidosis, metachromatic leucodystrophy
Malformations associated with increased fluid		Hydranencephaly Porencephaly – holoprosencephaly
Thickened skull		Bone marrow expansion – thalassaemia Bone expansion – rickets, osteogenesis imperfecta, osteopetrosis, cleidocranial dysostosis
Hypertensive		
Chronic hydrocephaly	Communicating	Previous intracranial bleed Meningitis Spina bifida Arnold–Chiari malformation
	Non-communicating	Aqueduct stenosis Dandy–Walker syndrome Periventricular haemorrhage
Chronic cerebral oedema		Benign intracranial hypertension Vitamin A intoxication
Chronic subdural effusion		Birth trauma Meningitis Child abuse Menkes syndrome

findings, I would suggest that he may have had an underlying congenital abnormality causing obstruction of CSF flow. This may take the form of congenital atresia of the aqueduct of Sylvius, or failure of formation of the foramina of Magendie and Luschka causing obstruction to flow at the outlet of the fourth ventricle.

MICROCEPHALY

STEM: Denise's parents are concerned that she is not doing what she should be doing at the age of 4 years. Please examine her.

PRESENTATION OF EXAMINATION FINDINGS

Denise is a 4-year-old girl with a small head relative to the rest of her body, although I would like to plot her head circumference, weight and height on a centile chart appropriate for her age and sex. She has no dysmorphic features and there are no shunts or reservoirs in situ. She appears to see and hear, although her vision and hearing should be formally tested. Her development is markedly delayed, in keeping with that of a 10-month-old child. I would like to measure the head circumference of both parents and to enquire about her birth history, with particular emphasis on mother's health before and during pregnancy and the delivery itself.

Thinking pause.....

Denise is a young girl with microcephaly and significantly delayed development. Damage to the developing brain either during pregnancy or at birth may account for this. She has no other features to suggest maternal rubella, alcohol abuse, or maternal hyperphenylalaninaemia.

How would you classify microcephaly?

1. Normal variation
2. Familial
3. Genetic – autosomal recessive, associated with learning difficulties
4. Secondary microcephaly:
   - perinatal (normal facies):
     — congenital infection – look for other signs
     — birth asphyxia – OFC normal at birth then falls off the centiles
   - fetal alcohol syndrome
   - syndromes associated with learning difficulties:
     — Cornelia de Lange
     — Rubinstein–Taybi
     — Smith–Lemli–Opitz

- syndromes associated with premature fusion of sutures (craniosynostosis):
  — Apert's
  — Crouzon's
  — Carpenter's
- Infant of mother with phenylketonuria

HEMIPLEGIA

STEM: This 4-year-old boy has always been weak down his right side. Please examine him.

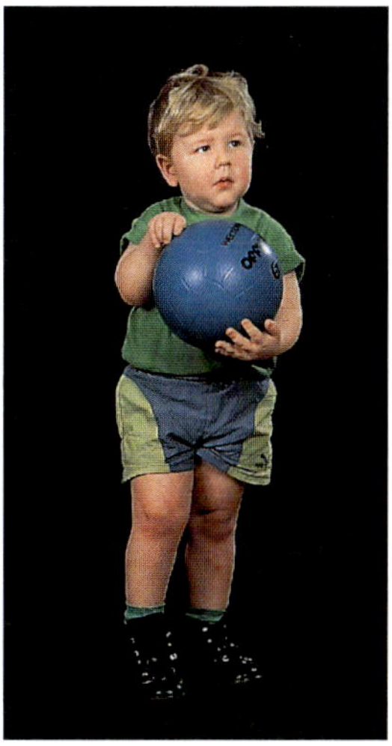

Fig. 5.2 *A child with a right spastic hemiplegia. His right arm is hyperpronated.* (Reproduced with kind permission from Lissauer T, Clayden G. Illustrated Textbook of Paediatrics, 2nd edn. Edinburgh: Mosby, 2001.)

PRESENTATION OF EXAMINATION FINDINGS

On walking he has a typical right-sided hemiplegic gait with flexed arm and extended leg and a secondary scoliosis. Paul is a boy with an abnormal posture at rest. He sits unsupported with his right arm flexed at the elbow and wrist, with his forearm pronated. He is wearing Piedro boots. The muscle bulk is reduced on his right side and he has increased tone in his right arm and leg with clonus of his right lower limb. The power is slightly reduced in his right side. In his upper limb the extensors are weaker than the arm flexors and in his leg his flexors are less powerful than the extensors. He has hyper-reflexia in both his right arm and leg. Sensation appears to be intact.

Thinking pause.....
This patient has a right-sided hemiplegia.

Anything else?

I would also like to examine his visual fields for a homonymous hemianopia, which would suggest a cortical lesion. It is also important to obtain a detailed birth history, history of epilepsy and perform a full developmental assessment.

What may have caused this?

About 50% are thought to be congenital and the other half, acquired. Of the congenital causes birth trauma is included along with antenatal insults. Strokes in childhood are fortunately rare and more commonly result from vascular occlusion than intracerebral haemorrhage beyond the neonatal period. Acquired hemiplegia is generally divided into the following groups:

Vascular lesions

- Trauma to head and neck vessels at birth, accidental hanging, falls on objects
- Arteritis and atherosclerosis are rare in children
- Metabolic diseases: abnormal vessels are found in Menkes disease, homocystinuria and Fabry's disease
- Mitochondrial disorders, e.g. MELAS syndrome
- Moya Moya disease: abnormal vessels in children with repeated strokes
- Vascular spasm: hemiplegic migraine

Thrombosis

- Hyperviscosity: polycythaemia can occur in neonate, cyanotic congenital heart disease, severe dehydration secondary to gastroenteritis, poorly controlled diabetes with persistent ketoacidosis, hyperlipidaemia, hyponatraemia and hyperviscosity
- Hypercoagulable states: DIC associated with sepsis, postsplenectomy, sickle cell disease, thalassaemia, protein, C and S and Factor V Leiden abnormalities.
- Embolization: congenital heart disease especially postsurgery.

Intracerebral haemorrhage

- Haemorrhagic disease of the newborn – probably the commonest cause of hemiplegia in term infant
- Grade IV periventricular haemorrhage in preterm infant
- Haemophilia
- Idiopathic thrombocytopenic purpura

Infection

- Haemophilus meningitis
- Viral encephalitis
- Abscess from middle ear infection

Trauma

- NAI
- Accidental injury, e.g. pressure from an extradural or subdural haematoma

Hypoxia

- Periventricular leucomalacia – commonest identified cause of hemiplegia in UK
- Birth asphyxia – in term infants
- Status epilepticus
- Head injury
- Cardiac arrest
- Acute hypotension from blood loss or endotoxic shock
- Generally associated with more widespread damage, ataxia, learning difficulties
- Dystonia, epilepsy with or without cortical blindness

Neoplasia

- Glioma (astrocytoma) Grade I–IV
- Primitive neuroectodermal tumour (PNET)

How would you manage a child with hemiplegia once the acute situation is over?

Management involves a multidisciplinary team approach to rehabilitation. Support involving physiotherapy, speech therapy, occupational therapy are generally required. Audiology and visual services may also be involved depending on the extent of the damage. Medical therapy may be necessary to control seizures and muscle spasms. Adequate footwear is essential. Once the child leaves hospital it is important to ensure that appropriate community care is organised. Such a child will be placed on the special needs system and thus reviewed regularly by the community paediatricians who will ensure that all the various support services are in place and also play a role in ensuring the child's education needs are adequately met.

DIPLEGIA

STEM: Jamie was born prematurely and is able to walk with the help of crutches. Please examine him.

PRESENTATION OF EXAMINATION FINDINGS

Jamie is a 15-year-old boy with increased tone, more so in his lower than upper limbs. In his upper limbs he has a spastic catch and demonstrates mild dyspraxia. He has normal power. His reflexes are generally brisk bilaterally with ankle clonus and extensor plantars. He has reduced range of movement at the ankles with tight Achilles tendons. On standing he has a flexed posture, being flexed at the hips and knees with equinus of the ankles. His legs are internally rotated at the hips. He normally walks with the aid of crutches but can walk independently over short distances and he has the classic waddling diplegic gait taking the weight on his toes. His speech is of normal quality and the content is appropriate for his age. His level of understanding seems in keeping with that of a 15 year old.

Thinking pause.....

Jamie is a teenage boy with a spastic diplegic cerebral palsy. I would like to know if there is a history of prematurity and low birth weight. I would also like to know how he performs at school and what support he requires. There is lack of evidence to suggest a genetic syndrome and no dysmorphic features associated with congenital infection or alcohol abuse. Given the pattern of spastic diplegia, with upper limb dyspraxia and apparently normal intelligence, the most likely underlying cause of diplegia is low birth weight. This type of cerebral palsy is known as Little's disease.

What is the natural course of this type of cerebral palsy?

This is characterised by a dystonic phase followed by the spastic stage of diplegia. During the dystonic phase the child shows marked extensor hypertonus, usually apparent from about 4 months of age onwards, with retention of primitive reflexes. This phase generally disappears by about 7–8 months of age and is followed by the spastic phase, associated with exaggerated tendon reflexes and the development of fixed flexion deformities. Less severely affected children learn to walk with the aid of a rotator or tripod and some can walk independently. These children are generally of normal intelligence and do not have epilepsy, but myopia with a degree of convergent squint and upper limb dyspraxia do occur. In later childhood 80% of the children will have a normal CT scan.

What is cerebral palsy?

It is a non-progressive disorder of motor and posture occurring as a result of damage to the developing brain.

What else may cause diplegia?

The causes of diplegic cerebral palsy can be divided into five groups as follows:

1. *Genetic causes*: associated with several syndromes, e.g. osteogenesis imperfecta, Pelizaeus–Merzbacher syndrome.
2. *Abnormalities of pregnancy*: brain damage selectively affecting the leg area, congenital infection, foetal alcohol syndrome, maternal phenylketonuria.
3. *Perinatal asphyxia*: in periventricular leucomalacia where the leg area is selectively affected as a watershed zone lesion – often associated with microcephaly, learning difficulties, behavioural difficulties and speech problems.
4. *Low birth weight*: as discussed. The aetiology is uncertain and appears to be some form of encephalopathy of low birth weight unrelated to subependymal haemorrhages, hyperbilirubinaemia, hypoglycaemia, hypoxia or birth trauma.
5. *Acquired causes*: sagittal sinus thrombosis in severe dehydration or hyperviscosity states.

VENTRICULOPERITONEAL SHUNT

STEM: Michael has had problems with hydrocephalus. Please examine him and tell us what you find.

PRESENTATION OF EXAMINATION FINDINGS

Michael is a 7-year-old boy with a large head and a ventriculoperitoneal shunt in situ. The reservoir is palpable in the right parietal area and the shunt can be felt postauricularly, down the right side of the neck, most probably ending in the peritoneum in view of the small scars in the right hypochondrium. He has an old non-functioning reservoir on the left parietal area and evidence of old abdominal scarring from previous peritoneal shunts. He has no papilloedema on fundoscopy. Neurological examination was normal.

Thinking pause.....

Michael is a young boy with two CSF access devices, one non-functioning and the other in connection with a ventriculoperitoneal shunt. He has no evidence of decompensated hydrocephalus. The underlying hydrocephaly may have been secondary to obstruction to CSF flow or, less likely, reduced CSF reabsorption. I would like to ask his parents if he was born prematurely, and if so, was there any history of intraventricular haemorrhage. Shunting may have been required for posthaemorrhagic hydrocephalus.

What are the complications of CSF shunting?

Complications depend upon the type of shunting device used. The most common management of hydrocephalus is to use a ventriculoperitoneal shunt and separate CSF access device, which allows direct measurement of intracranial pressure, reducing the number of unnecessary shunt revisions. Mechanical problems may arise from blockage of the shunt, fracture or migration of the tubing. Blockage by choroid plexus, fibrin, blood clot and brain fragments may cause raised intracranial pressure. More commonly distal blocking occurs due to pocketing of CSF from adhesions, preventing CSF flow through the peritoneum. Infection does occur and intrathecal and intravenous antibiotics are used as first line treatment of ventriculitis followed by shunt replacement if necessary.

Other rare complications include slit ventricle syndrome, intestinal obstruction (volvulus), peritonitis and peritoneal fibrosis.

What is slit ventricle syndrome?

This occurs following overdrainage, either from acute or chronic CSF decompression. It is characterised by three components:

1. an intermittent or chronic headache secondary to ventricular catheter obstruction

2. slit-like, Y shaped ventricles as seen on CT scan
3. the valve mechanism is slow to refill.

Management of this condition has involved several procedures, including use of high-pressure valves, steroids and head-down position, and an antisiphon valve has been developed.

What is the prognosis for patients with hydrocephalus?

Epilepsy is reported to occur in up to 50% of patients in some studies, although usually significantly less. The frontal lobe is one of the most epileptogenic regions of the brain and there is a risk of precipitating seizures from frontal reservoirs. Hemiplegia has also been reported to occur, secondary to hydrocephalus, either due to the underlying aetiology, such as meningitis, or as a complication of the hydrocephalus, such as shunt insertion involving the motor cortex or subdural haemorrhage from overdrainage. Vision may be impaired for a number of reasons, e.g. the development of optic atrophy, compression of the optic chiasm or posterior cerebral artery. Intelligence is generally normal in half to two-thirds of patients with shunted hydrocephalus.

CSF ACCESS DEVICE

STEM: Please observe this 10-week-old girl and tell us what you notice.

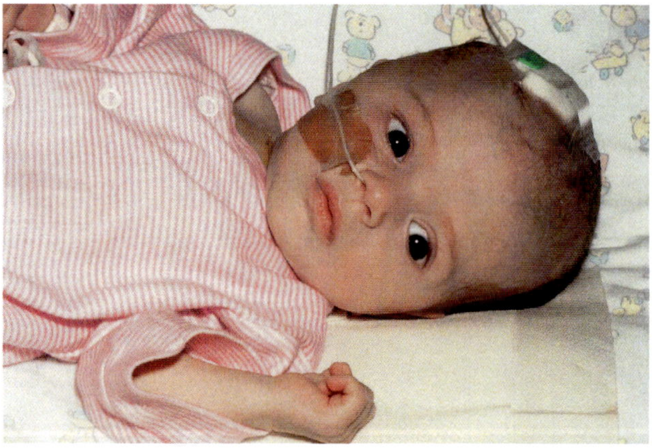

Fig. 5.3 *CSF access device.*

PRESENTATION OF EXAMINATION FINDINGS

Sophie is a 10-week-old girl with a nasogastric tube in situ and a butterfly needle sited in a CSF access device (Rickham reservoir). She is pink and well perfused and does not look dysmorphic but appears very thin for her age. I would like to perform a full neurodevelopmental examination.

Thinking pause.....

This is an infant with a CSF access device which may be a consequence of having had raised intracranial pressure or hydrocephalus. I would like to obtain further history.

Further history

Sophie presented with a history of intermittent vomiting and failure to thrive.

What further investigations might be helpful?

A cerebral ultrasound scan in an infant who has an open anterior fontanelle would be helpful.

The cerebral ultrasound scan showed hydrocephalus and raised a strong suspicion of a central midline brain tumour, which was confirmed on MRI imaging.

What clinical features might you expect to find on examination?

A 10-week-old baby with hydrocephalus is likely to have an increased head circumference which I would like to measure and plot on the appropriate centile chart together with her weight and length. There may be dilated scalp veins, sunsetting of the eyes, irritability and problems with feeding and weight gain. She may develop a VIth nerve palsy.

What treatment options are available for a small infant with a large brain tumour?

Brain tumours in infants are rare and a biopsy, if the neurosurgeon thought it was safe, would be required to formally make the diagnosis. Possibilities include malignant astrocytoma, ependymoma, atypical teratoid/rhabdoid tumour, medulloblastoma. The real problem with infants with brain tumours is that they are not suitable candidates for cranial radiotherapy as part of their treatment. The effect on normal brain tissue is too damaging and the neurodevelopmental outcome extremely poor. Current management of an infant with a brain tumour includes a surgical diagnosis and excision, if at all possible, followed by intensive chemotherapy. The plan would be to continue chemotherapy for as long as possible so that radiotherapy can be avoided until at least the age of 3 years.

This baby has a CSF access device. What problems are associated with it?

The main problem is the risk of infection when the CSF access device is tapped.

What are the advantages of a CSF access device?

It allows measurement of intraventricular pressure and analysis of CSF fluid for evidence of infection. It has now become fairly common practice for CSF access devices to be inserted at around the same time as ventriculoperitoneal shunts for the management of hydrocephalus in many units.

Are parents who have had a child with a brain tumour at increased likelihood of having another child with a brain tumour?

This is a difficult question but the occurrence of a second child with a tumour in the family is around 1% apart from in inherited retinoblastoma and in the Li–Fraumeni syndrome, known as family cancer syndrome, where there is an inherited abnormality of the p53 tumour suppresser gene.

ERB'S PALSY

STEM: This baby had a very difficult delivery. Please examine him.

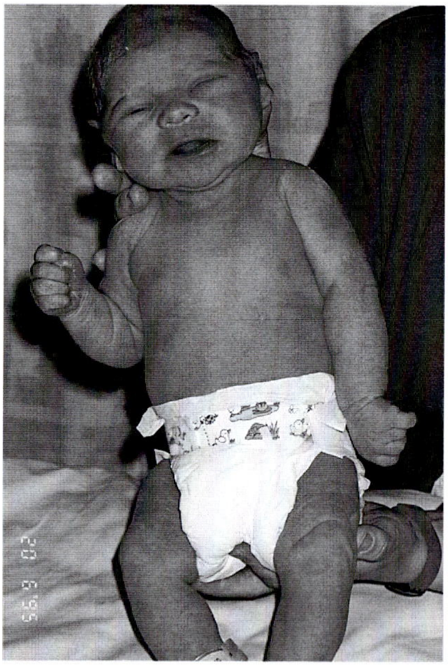

Fig. 5.4 *Extended and pronated posture of the affected left arm in Erb's palsy.* (Reproduced with kind permission from Johnston P, Flood K, Spinks K. The Newborn Child, 9th edn. Edinburgh: Churchill Livingstone, 2003.)

PRESENTATION OF EXAMINATION FINDINGS

Geoff is a large baby with reduced tone and power in his left arm. His forearm is pronated and his wrist flexed, in the classical 'waiter's tip' position. His finger movements and grasp reflex are normal but his left biceps reflex is absent and Moro reflex is asymmetrical. He has no other neurological abnormalities.

Thinking pause.....
This is a baby with Erb's palsy. I would like to ask his parents whether he was a breech presentation or if there was shoulder dystocia.

Where is the underlying lesion?

The clinical picture results from damage to the upper brachial plexus root, C5 and C6, during delivery causing paralysis of the deltoid, brachioradialis and long wrist extensor muscles.

What advice would you give to the parents?

I would reassure the parents that this is not a permanent condition, but one that results from stretching of the nerves supplying some of the muscles of the arm and once the nerves heal Geoff will regain the use of his arm. I would explain that recovery is usually within 3 weeks (although if the injury is severe, it can take up to 2 years). I would arrange for the parents to be seen by the physiotherapist in order to teach them some passive limb exercises, and I would make an appointment to review Geoff in 3–4 weeks time.

PLAGIOCEPHALY

STEM: This 10-month-old boy's parents are worried about the shape of his head. What do you think?

PRESENTATION OF EXAMINATION FINDINGS

Jack is a 10-month-old boy with an asymmetrically shaped cranium, with mild flattening of the forehead and elevation of the orbit on the left side, with a minor degree of frontal prominence on the right side. I would like to plot his head circumference, length and weight on a growth chart appropriate for his age and sex, although his head does not appear obviously disproportionately large to the other parameters. Jack has no other dysmorphic features and no obvious abnormal neurology. He is able to sit unaided, transfer small objects, and has a neat pincer grip. He turns to sounds and says 'ma'.

Thinking pause.....
Jack is an infant with a mild degree of plagiocephaly due to synostosis of the left coronal suture.

How does this differ from other types of synostosis?

Plagiocephaly is unilateral synostosis usually affecting the coronal suture. It is generally mild, common in early infancy and improves with time and is likely to be of no significance. More severe craniosynostosis with fusion of multiple or all sutures can occur resulting in microcephaly with associated raised intracranial pressure, mental retardation and other neurological sequelae. These may be congenital, e.g. Apert's or Crouzon's syndromes, or acquired after metabolic disorders, such as idiopathic hypercalcaemia.

FRIEDREICH'S ATAXIA

STEM: Caroline is very unsteady on her feet and is described as being clumsy. Please examine her neurologically.

PRESENTATION OF EXAMINATION FINDINGS

Caroline is a 15-year-old girl with incoordination of her limbs and gait. She has decreased tone and her power is reduced in her lower limbs bilaterally. There is a mild degree of distal limb muscle wasting present. Her knee and ankle reflexes are absent but she has extensor plantar responses and has pes cavus. She also demonstrates loss of position and vibration sense. Caroline has an intention tremor with past pointing and dysdiadochokinesis. She also has nystagmus and moderate dysarthria. She walks with an unsteady broad-based gait and on general observation I note that she has a degree of kyphoscoliosis.

Thinking pause.....

The most likely diagnosis is Friedreich's ataxia. I would also like to look for optic atrophy and to examine the cardiovascular system.

How is this condition inherited?

Inheritance is autosomal recessive and the gene locus is on chromosome 9. It generally presents with progressive clumsiness.

What is the underlying pathology?

The main pathology is in the spinal cord with demyelination and degeneration of the posterior columns, corticospinal pathways and spinocerebellar tracts. As the inheritance is autosomal recessive it is believed to be a consequence of an underlying metabolic disorder, probably of carbohydrate metabolism. This is based on the observation that inhibitors of various Krebs cycle enzymes, such as pyruvate dehydrogenase or pyruvate decarboxylase, are associated with various types of progressive ataxia.

What is the prognosis for this condition?

Various diets have been tried unsuccessfully, based on possible biochemical aetiology. Treatment is largely supportive. With progressive ataxia most patients are wheelchair-bound by their mid-twenties and death occurs at 40–50 years of age due to cardiorespiratory complications. Scoliosis develops in more than 75% of cases and if severe can cause death from secondary cardiorespiratory embarrassment. Cardiac abnormalities, particularly hypertrophic cardiomyopathy, may present with angina or arrhythmias, and murmurs may suggest papillary muscle rupture or left ventricular outlet obstruction.

ATAXIC TELANGIECTASIA

STEM: This 9-year-old girl has been slow to develop skills and has poor balance. Please examine her neurologically.

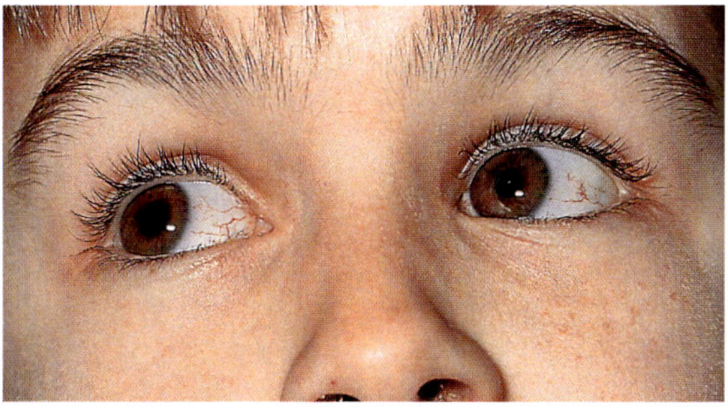

Fig. 5.5 *Telangiectasia of the conjunctiva are present from about 4 years of age in ataxic telangiectasia.*
(Reproduced with kind permission from Lissauer T, Clayden G. Illustrated Textbook of Paediatrics, 2nd edn. Edinburgh: Mosby, 2001.)

PRESENTATION OF EXAMINATION FINDINGS

Maurvin is a 9-year-old girl with telangiectasia of the conjunctiva, cheeks and ears. She has nystagmus and mild ophthalmoplegia with poor conjugate gaze. Her speech is dysarthric and her behaviour is a little immature for her age. She has reduced muscle tone and poor coordination but her power is normal. Her plantar reflexes are flexor and proprioception and vibration sense are intact. Her gait is unsteady and broad based. She has no cutaneous patches of hypopigmentation or hyperpigmentation, or dermatitis. I would like to plot her height and weight on a growth chart appropriate for her age and sex, as she appears to be relatively short for her age.

Thinking pause.....
Maurvin has evidence of spinocerebellar degeneration with facial telangiectasia and a degree of developmental delay. The most likely diagnosis is ataxic telangiectasia. I would like to ask her parents about her developmental milestones, as there is often motor delay in infancy, and to ask about school performance. These children are susceptible to infection and have an increased risk of developing non-Hodgkin's lymphoma.

How would you confirm the diagnosis?
The diagnosis is a clinical one, but other indicators are low IgA levels and occasionally IgG_2 and IgG_4 and IgE, in up to 70%, and elevated serum α-fetoprotein. Eosinophilia may be present.

How is this condition inherited?
Inheritance is autosomal recessive and the gene defect is located on chromosome 11.

What problems is it associated with?
Thymic hypoplasia results in abnormal T-cells and consequently infections are common due to abnormal cellular immunity and to low immunoglobulin levels. There is a 50–100-fold increased risk of malignancy, due to a defect in DNA repair mechanisms, particularly lymphoreticular tumours, such as non-Hodgkin's lymphoma.

How are these children managed?
Control of recurrent infections is essential, as is minimizing exposure to radiation. The latter obviously has important implications for screening and subsequent treatment of malignancies. Progression of ataxia and choreoathetosis usually means that most children are wheelchair-bound by adolescence and death usually occurs before adulthood.

HEREDITARY MOTOR AND SENSORY NEUROPATHY

STEM: This 7-year-old boy has difficulties with walking. Please examine him.

PRESENTATION OF EXAMINATION FINDINGS

Joshua is a 7-year-old boy with wasting of the distal muscles of the lower limbs and pes cavus. He has distal sensory loss and diminished reflexes. He walks with a 'steppage' foot drop ataxic gait.

Thinking pause.....
Joshua is a young boy with a peripheral motor and sensory neuropathy.

What is the underlying pathology?
This group of peripheral nerve disorders is due to demyelination and remyelination of the peripheral nerves resulting in hypertrophy of the nerves, which show a characteristic 'onion bulb formation' on biopsy. Several types exist and they can be inherited in an autosomal dominant or autosomal recessive form of the disease. The autosomal dominant form of Type I is due to a defective gene located on chromosome 1 and was

previously known as peroneal muscular atrophy or Charcot–Marie–Tooth disease.

DUCHENNE MUSCULAR DYSTROPHY

STEM: This 6-year-old boy seems to his parents to be weaker generally and is now having difficulty climbing the stairs. Please examine him.

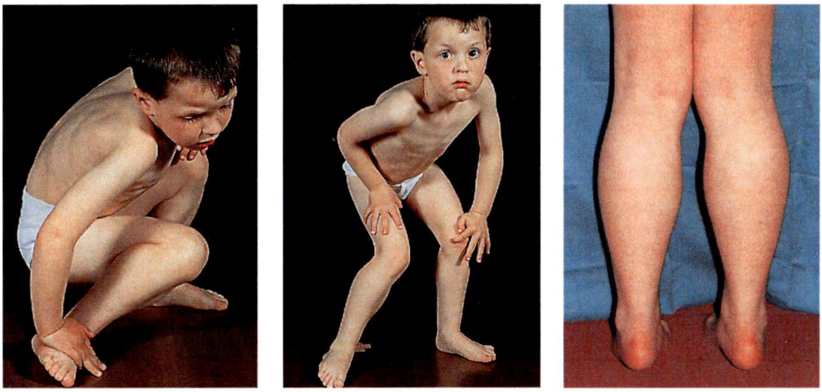

a b c

Fig. 5.6 **(a, b)** *Gower's sign. The child needs to turn prone to rise, then uses his hands to climb up on his knees before standing, because of poor hip girdle fixation and/or proximal muscle weakness. Any child continuing to do this after 3 years of age is likely to have a neuromuscular condition.* **(c)** *Hypertrophied calf muscles in Duchenne muscular dystrophy.*

(*a, b* Reproduced with kind permission from Lissauer T, Clayden G. Illustrated Textbook of Paediatrics, 2nd edn. Edinburgh: Mosby, 2001; *c*, Reproduced with kind permission from Thomas R, Harvey D. Paediatrics: Colour Guide. Edinburgh: Churchill Livingstone, 1997.)

PRESENTATION OF EXAMINATION FINDINGS

Peter is a 6-year-old boy with hypertrophy of his calf muscles and proximal muscle weakness. He walks with a waddling gait on his toes and stands with a lumbar lordosis. He does not yet have true tightening of the Achilles tendons, suggesting that the toe walking is necessary to compensate for the hip flexion contractures and lordosis. He rises from the floor by climbing up his legs, known as Gower's sign.

Thinking pause.....

This is a young boy with Duchenne muscular dystrophy (DMD).

How would you confirm the diagnosis?

Creatinine phosphokinase (CPK) is grossly elevated in the early stages of the disease and electromyography is usually abnormal. Definitive diagnosis is with muscle biopsy, which shows a characteristic appearance. DNA studies can also be done to look for the dystrophin gene.

How is this condition inherited?

DMD is a sex-linked recessive disorder with the lesion of the dystrophin gene on the short arm of the X chromosome in the region of Xp21. DMD can occur in females with Turner's syndrome and may occur in a milder form due to lyonisation. Approximately one-third of cases represent a new mutation. Antenatal diagnosis is possible.

How are these patients managed?

There is no cure for this condition and management is largely supportive. Regular physical exercise is encouraged to prevent muscle contractures, especially of the hip flexors and Achilles tendons. As the muscle is replaced by fat the children may become obese and dietary advice is necessary to aid mobilization in the early years. Ambulation can be maintained using orthosis and surgery to release contractures but all children will eventually require a wheelchair, usually by the age of 10–14 years. Once the child is wheelchair-bound, scoliosis develops with consequent reduction in vital capacity and surgery is often required. Almost one-third of children have learning difficulties but all children should be supported educationally as success at school will give them a sense of achievement.

What is the prognosis for this condition?

Chest deformity and distortion of the diaphragm may result in oesophageal reflux, oesophagitis and haematemesis with increased risk of aspiration pneumonia. Cor pulmonale develops due to chest deformities and cardiac muscle involvement usually results in cardiorespiratory failure and death by the early twenties.

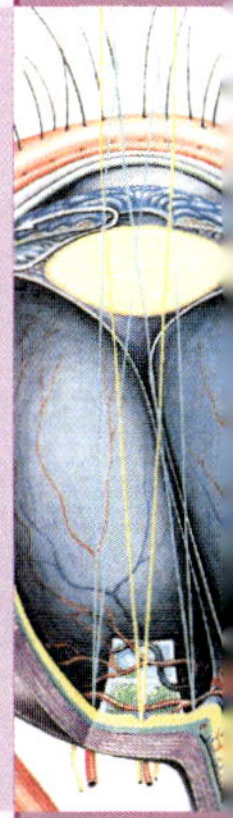

6
EYES

Candidates are frequently asked to examine the patient's eyes in the exam as a number of conditions make good cases for the exam and are often readily available. It is therefore important that you have given consideration to the most commonly encountered cases and practised a routine for the examination. You will rarely be expected to perform every aspect of the eye examination, although this is summarised below.

SUMMARY OF EXAMINATION OF THE EYES

Always start by checking whether the child can see out of both eyes

INSPECTION

- Ptosis, nystagmus, strabismus, cataracts, pupil size inequality
- Structural anomaly: exophthalmos, endophthalmos, eyelid defects, coloboma, craniosynostosis

PUPILS

Red reflexes

Pupillary reflexes: direct light reflex, consensual light reflex, accommodation

1. Large pupils:
   - — sympathomimetics
   - — alcohol
   - — Holmes–Adie – large, reacts slowly to light
   - — ocular blindness – consensual response in other eye, nil from affected eye
   - — cortical blindness – no response to light but reacts to accommodation
2. Small pupils:
   - — opiates
   - — Horner's syndrome
   - — Argyll Robertson (very rare even in adults)

VISUAL ACUITY

Depends on age of child:

- 4 weeks – fix on parent's face, VEP, Catford Drum, preferential looking tests
- 6 weeks – follow object 90 cm away through 90° (not to midline)
- 3 months – follow object at 90 cm through 180° when supine
- 10 months – picks up raisins with pincer grip, test with each eye covered (may need to cover eye with a patch)
- 1 year – picks up hundreds and thousands
- 2–3 years – miniature toys – use seven known toys and ask 'What's this?'; test each eye
- 3 years – Stycar matching letters at 3 m and near
- 5 years – Snellen charts

EYE MOVEMENTS

VISUAL FIELDS

1. Confrontation perimetry:
   - test each eye separately and then both together to exclude sensory inattention; don't forget to test for scotomata
2. Defects:
   - concentric decrease – retinitis pigmentosa
   - central scotoma – macular lesions, benign and pathological ICP
   - bitemporal hemianopia – craniopharyngioma
   - homonymous hemianopia – optic tract lesion
   - quadrantianopia – upper: lower fibres in temporal radiation lesion ± speech; lower: upper fibres in parietal radiation

TEST FOR STRABISMUS

Cover/uncover test

FUNDOSCOPY

Begin with ophthalmoscope at +12 dioptres (red numbers) and gradually adjust it until you can focus on the retina. Look at:

- Cornea – corneal abrasions
- Lens – cataracts
- Disc – optic atrophy, papilloedema, glaucoma
- Arteries – know grading of hypertension
- Retina – exudates, haemorrhages, retinitis pigmentosa

SHORT CASES FOR EYE CONDITIONS

BENIGN INTRACRANIAL HYPERTENSION

STEM: Please examine Sharon's eyes. She has bad headaches and is sometimes sick in the morning.

PRESENTATION OF EXAMINATION FINDINGS

Sharon is an overweight teenage girl with papilloedema on fundoscopy. She has no retinal haemorrhages or changes suggesting hypertensive retinopathy and her blood pressure is normal. Confrontation perimetry is normal but she has bilateral central scotomata. Her vision is a little blurred on distance testing but otherwise the neurological examination is entirely normal.

Thinking pause.....

The most likely diagnosis in this setting would be benign intracranial hypertension.

How would you confirm the diagnosis?

I would want to perform a CT scan to exclude a space-occupying lesion and hydrocephalus. A lumbar puncture should be performed to measure the CSF pressure.

What is the cause of BIH?

There are numerous causes for this including haematological conditions, endocrine causes, drugs, trauma, infections and other systemic conditions, although in 50% of the cases the cause is unknown. The exact pathophysiology is uncertain but the most popular theory is decreased CSF absorption.

How would you manage this patient?

BIH is generally a self-limiting condition although various measures can be used to reduce intracranial pressure. Reduction in CSF volume by repeated removal at daily lumbar punctures can be tried but this temporary measure represents an unpleasant ordeal, requiring sedation. Corticosteroid treatment with dexamethasone has been shown in a few reports to reduce pressure but this has not been substantiated. For patients in whom steroids are unsuccessful, acetazolamide can be used either alone or, more commonly, with a loop diuretic. If medical treatment fails a ventriculoperitoneal or lumboperitoneal shunt can be inserted, with good results. Very rarely optic nerve decompression may be required to relieve symptoms.

BITEMPORAL HEMIANOPIA

STEM: Stephen's parents have noticed that he has a tendency to bump into things. They are also concerned that he is the smallest in his class at school. Please examine his eyes.

PRESENTATION OF EXAMINATION FINDINGS

Stephen is a 10-year-old boy who appears short and relatively overweight. He has bitemporal hemianopia on visual field testing by confrontation. His discs are pale but there is no papilloedema present. The remainder of the cranial nerves are intact and I would like to do a full neurological examination. I would also like to plot his height and weight on a growth chart appropriate for his age and sex. I would like to ask specifically about symptoms of diabetes insipidus and hypothyroidism although he has no clinical evidence of thyroid disease.

Thinking pause.....

Stephen is a boy with bitemporal hemianopia, which may be secondary to a space-occupying lesion compressing the optic chiasma, the most likely cause being a craniopharyngioma.

How would you confirm your diagnosis?

Plain lateral skull X-ray is often diagnostic in revealing a calcified mass eroding the clinoid process with an abnormally enlarged sella. The diagnosis, and any suprasellar extension, can be confirmed by CT or MRI. Assessment of pituitary function will also be necessary.

How is this condition managed?

Surgical resection is indicated if there are visual or neurological disturbances. Between 75 and 80% of patients can have their tumours debulked with a recurrence rate of 20–25%. Steroids can be used preoperatively to reduce pressure and vasopressin used to control diabetes insipidus. Hormone deficiencies should be corrected and hydrocortisone is always required for the stress of surgical procedures even if ACTH levels are normal. Long-term follow-up with CT scanning, endocrine function and vision testing are necessary to monitor the efficacy of treatment.

What is the prognosis for this condition?

Craniopharyngioma should be considered to be a chronic condition. If there is no evidence of disease or calcification on CT scan there is an estimated 70% 10-year survival rate. If residual tumour or calcification remains after surgery, then radiotherapy may be indicated. There is no role for chemotherapy at present.

PTOSIS

STEM: Emma is concerned that her eyelids are droopy. She is quite anxious and everything is exhausting. Please examine her neurologically.

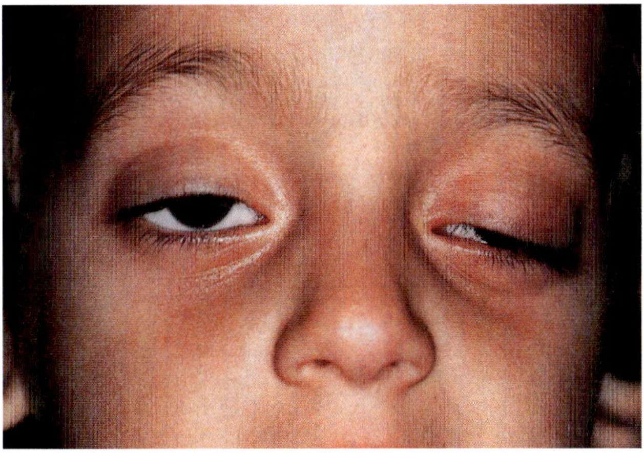

Fig. 6.1 *Ptosis in myasthenia gravis.*
(Reproduced with kind permission from Thomas R, Harvey D. Paediatrics: Colour Guide. Edinburgh: Churchill Livingstone, 1997.)

PRESENTATION OF EXAMINATION FINDINGS

Emma is a 13-year-old girl with bilateral partial ptosis. She has normal pupillary reflexes and eye movements are diminished. On repeated blinking exercises she demonstrates ocular muscle fatiguability with increasing ptosis. She also has reduced facial expression. She has difficulty making hair-brushing movements and is slow to stand from a crouched position. Climbing stairs is also difficult.

Thinking pause.....

Emma demonstrates weakness of ocular muscles and proximal muscle weakness with abnormal muscle fatiguability after repeated activity, suggesting a diagnosis of myasthenia gravis. Due to her age this is likely to be the juvenile form, which is similar to the adult autoimmune type and is associated with high titres or antibody to the acetylcholine receptor.

How would you confirm the diagnosis?

Diagnosis is made by observing an improvement following administration of edrophonium (Tensilon). Muscle fatiguability can be demonstrated by stimulating the peripheral nerve using surface electrodes at 4 or 10 Hz.

How would you manage this patient?

Medical treatment is with anticholinesterases such as neostigmine or pyridostigmine. In the longer term immunosuppressive therapy with carefully tailored alternate day prednisolone or azathioprine may be required to maintain remission. In the emergency situation plasma exchange may be required for crisis if there is respiratory paralysis or bulbar paralysis. If a thymoma is present or the response to medical therapy is poor, thymectomy may be performed.

What are the causes of ptosis?

Causes of ptosis are as outlined in Table 6.1.

Table 6.1 Causes of ptosis

Type of ptosis	Cause	Related condition
Unilateral	IIIrd nerve palsy complete/incomplete (partial) (fixed dilated pupil, eye down and out)	Posterior communicating artery aneurysm Suprasellar tumour Ophthalmoplegic migraine Orbit lesion Cavernous sinus thrombosis Midbrain tumour
	Horner's syndrome (partial ptosis)	Congenital – heterochromia iridae Neuroblastoma with lung apex/ cervical sympathetic chain involved Postcardiac surgery – look for thoracic scar Klumpke's paralysis Brainstem tumour
Bilateral	Congenital Myasthenia gravis Myopathy	Wrinkling forehead, fatiguability

NYSTAGMUS

STEM: Darren has always had jerky eye movements. Please examine his eyes.

PRESENTATION OF EXAMINATION FINDINGS

Darren is a 4-year-old boy with bilateral horizontal nystagmus. The intensity of the nystagmus is equal on both sides and is independent of the direction of gaze. He has normal vision. Darren also has normal cerebellar function and the remainder of the neurological examination is normal.

Thinking pause.....
In this well boy with no other signs the most likely diagnosis is congenital nystagmus. I would also like to check his hearing and ocular fundi.

What is 'congenital' nystagmus?

It is isolated nystagmus of unknown cause and is sometimes familial. The condition may improve with age.

Causes of nystagmus

Nystagmus describes involuntary oscillations of the eye, which may be horizontal, vertical or rotatory (Table 6.2). It is defined by the fast phase, but it is the slow phase which is pathological, other than pendular nystagmus, where there is no fast phase. Nystagmus may be caused by pathology in the brainstem, cerebellum, cervical cord or inner ear.

Table 6.2 Causes of nystagmus

Type of nystagmus	Features	Related condition
Ocular	Pendular/rotatory	Oculocutaneous albinism Congenital – poor visual acuity Blindness
Central	Nystagmus in any direction 1. Up-beat 2. Down-beat	Brainstem lesion e.g. vertebrobasilar ischaemia Lesion in floor of fourth ventricle, pontine tegmentum Extrinsic compressive lesion of foramen magnum
Cerebellar		Fast phase is towards side of lesion
Vestibular		Unidirectional – away from side of lesion
Positional		Unidirectional Benign positional vertigo Head injury Postviral labyrinthitis

SQUINT

STEM: Eilidh is a 6-year-old girl whose parents are worried that there is something wrong with her eyes, particularly after school in the evenings. Please examine her eyes.

PRESENTATION OF EXAMINATION FINDINGS

Eilidh is a 6-year-old girl with misalignment of the visual axis, which is normally corrected by wearing glasses. Her right eye turns inwards at rest when her glasses are removed. The angle subtended by the eyes does not vary with the direction of the gaze. The cover test confirms the presence of a manifest right-sided strabismus. She appears to have impaired near vision with intact distance vision, although more formal testing is required to assess the extent of the refractive error. Her optic fundi are normal.

Thinking pause.....
Eilidh has a concomitant (non-paralytic) manifest squint secondary to a hypermetropic refractive error.

When would you worry about squints in an infant?
Any infant with a fixed squint or any squint persisting beyond 2 months of age should be referred to a specialist paediatric ophthalmologist for further assessment. Although squints are most commonly due to failure to develop binocular vision due to a refractive error, cataracts, retinoblastoma and other intraocular causes must be excluded. Prevention of amblyopia is essential and refractive errors are corrected with glasses.

Table 6.3 Causes of squint*

Type of squint	Features	Causes and resulting condition
Non-paralytic (concomitant)	Deviation unchanged in all directions Common Convergent (85%) or divergent Usually horizontal (rarely vertical)	Refractive error: amblyopia, hypermetropia, anisometropia Eye disease (often divergent): corneal scar, cataract, optic atrophy, retinal disease Failure to develop normal binocular vision: usually congenital
Paralytic	Deviation varies with direction of gaze Rare	Extraocular muscle palsy: III – divergent squint; IV/VI – convergent squint Extraocular muscle weakness: myopathies, Duane's syndrome, Brown's syndrome
Pseudosquint	Common in children, tends to disappear with facial development Confirmed by negative cover test	Marked epicanthic folds Small or large interpupillary distance Broad nasal bridge Facial asymmetry

* Abnormal if more than 6 months old.

Types and causes of squint (abnormal if more than 6 months old) are shown in Table 6.3.

What are the cover tests?

There are two types of test used to assess a squint:

1. *Cover/uncover test*: one eye is covered and the other is observed. If the uncovered eye moves to fix upon the object there is a squint, which is present all the time – a manifest squint. Each eye is tested in turn.
2. *Alternate cover test*: if the cover/uncover test is normal, excluding a manifest squint, this test is used. The occluder is moved to and fro between the eyes and if the eye which has been uncovered moves then a latent squint is present.

LENS DISLOCATION

STEM: Robbie is a 15-year-old boy who is the tallest in his class. Please examine him.

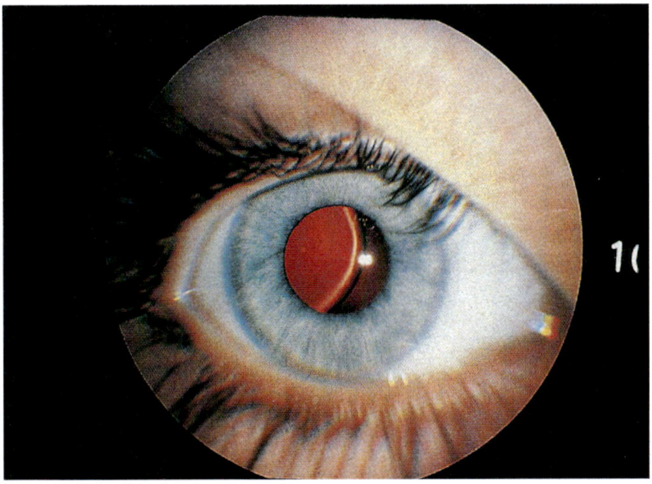

Fig. 6.2 *Lens subluxation. In Marfan's syndrome the lens is dislocated laterally upwards and outwards.*
(Reproduced with kind permission from Campbell AGM, McIntosh N (eds) Forfar & Arneil's Textbook of Pediatrics, 4th edn. Edinburgh: Churchill Livingstone, 1992.)

PRESENTATION OF EXAMINATION FINDINGS

Robbie is a tall 15-year-old boy with glasses and a marfinoid appearance. Examination of vision reveals severe myopia and he has upward and outward subluxation of his right lens. There is no evidence of retinal detachment or cataracts, although more formal assessment by a specialist ophthalmologist would be required. In addition he has a high arched palate and long thin fingers. The lower segment of his body is longer than the upper segment and his arm span is greater than his height. His joints are hyperextensible.

Thinking pause.....
Robbie is a 15-year-old boy with Marfan's syndrome and subluxation of his right lens. I would also like to examine his chest for evidence of scoliosis and listen to his heart for murmurs suggestive of aortic or mitral valve disease.

Could the underlying condition be homocystinuria?
Although both conditions have a similar phenotype, homocystinuria is associated with downward and inward lens subluxation, in contrast to the upward and outward subluxation found in Marfan's syndrome.

How is the diagnosis made?
Diagnosis is essentially clinical, although slit lamp examination and echocardiography are useful. Plasma urinary amino acids can be checked to exclude homocystinuria. Inheritance of Marfan's syndrome is autosomal dominant and if the diagnosis is uncertain, referral to a clinical geneticist is advisable, when a family tree can be drawn and gene studies undertaken to confirm a gene defect on chromosome 15.

OCULOCUTANEOUS ALBINISM

STEM: Jamila has always had jerky eye movements. What do you think may be the cause?

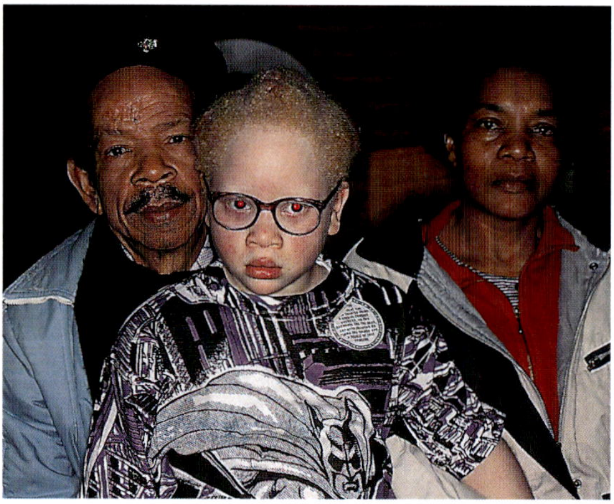

Fig. 6.3 *A child with oculocutaneous albinism with her parents.*
(Reproduced with kind permission from Lissauer T, Clayden G. Illustrated Textbook of Paediatrics, 2nd edn. Edinburgh: Mosby, 2001.)

PRESENTATION OF EXAMINATION FINDINGS

Jamila is an 8-year-old girl with depigmentation of the skin, hair and eyes. She lacks pigment in the iris, retina, eyelids and eyebrows. Jamila has pendular nystagmus and photophobia. She wears glasses and her visual acuity is severely impaired.

Thinking pause.....

Jamila is a young girl with oculocutaneous albinism.

What is albinism?

Albinism refers to a group of inherited disorders of the melanin pigment system in which there is a congenital reduction or an absence of melanin formation. Depending on the distribution of depigmentation in the skin and the eye the albinism may be oculocutaneous, ocular or partial. Types of albinism not associated with metabolic disorders include all types of oculocutaneous and ocular albinisms and are autosomal recessive, except for albinism, ocular late onset-sensorineural deafness, X-linked. Types of albinism associated with metabolic defects include the Albinism, oculocutaneous, Hermansky–Pudlak type and Chediak–Higashi syndrome.

All types of albinism are thought to result from different mutations involving the biosynthesis of melanin and are most probably due to an enzyme abnormality. The only enzyme shown to produce albinism when deficient is tyrosinase, which is low or absent in a number of types including tyrosinase negative, minimal pigment type and yellow mutant types of oculocutaneous albinism and in most cases of Hermansky–Pudlak type. However, tyrosinase activity is normal in all other types of oculocutaneous and ocular albinism.

The presence of ocular features is constant and is necessary to make a diagnosis of albinism and is characterised by foveal hypoplasia with an associated reduction in visual acuity that cannot be corrected to normal. Nystagmus is also a constant feature of albinism and usually presents within the first year of life.

How would you manage this patient?

Regular ophthalmological care is essential. Failure to develop the fixation reflex results from lack of eye pigment. There is no treatment but correction of refractive errors and fitting of tinted lenses from early infancy may allow normal fixation to develop. Children are prone to sunburn and skin cancer and protection with sun-hats and sunscreen is essential in bright sunlight. Genetic counselling is also advised.

What is the prognosis for this condition?

This group of disorders is associated with a normal life span except in the case of oculocutaneous albinism, Hermansky–Pudlak type, which is associated with a bleeding diathesis due to storage pool-deficient platelets, and death may result from haemorrhage.

HORNER'S SYNDROME

STEM: Laura has developed a droopy right eyelid. Please examine her eyes and tell us what you find.

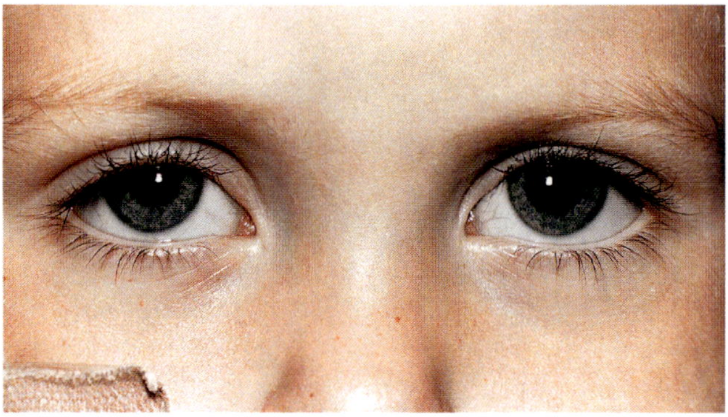

Fig. 6.4 *A girl with Horner's syndrome showing partial ptosis of her right eye with a myotic right pupil.*

PRESENTATION OF EXAMINATION FINDINGS

Laura is a 2-year-old pale, slim girl with a partial right-sided ptosis. Her right pupil is smaller in diameter than her left pupil but both pupils react to light and accommodation. There is no obvious exophthalmos and her external ocular movements are normal. She has near and distance vision in both eyes but I would like her to have more formal visual testing. She has lost her hair and has an indwelling central venous access device. She has no apical chest scars.

Thinking pause.....
Laura is a young girl with right-sided Horner's syndrome.

What is the likely cause of this in her case?

From Laura's appearance I would diagnose that she is having chemotherapy treatment for an underlying malignancy. I would predict that the site of the tumour is intrathoracic at the upper part of her thorax on the right-hand side, with consequent neuropraxis of the sympathetic distribution to her eye. It is possible that there is a mass higher up the neurological pathway causing compression at the level of the spinal cord, cerebellum or brainstem.

Causes of Horner's syndrome

- Congenital – heterochromia iridae
- Neuroblastoma with lung apex/cervical sympathetic chain
- Postcardiac surgery – look for thoracic scar

- Klumpke's paralysis
- Brainstem tumour.

PUPILLARY REFLEXES

STEM: Please examine this 4-year-old girl's eyes.

PRESENTATION OF EXAMINATION FINDINGS

Isla is a 4-year-old girl with pupillary size inequality and abnormal pupillary reflexes. She has no structural anomaly of her eyes and both irises are the same colour. Her left pupil is larger than the right and is unreactive to direct light and consensual light stimulation. The right eye has a normal direct light reflex but it is not possible to elicit a consensual reflex. The left eye has no ocular movements and Isla is blind in her left eye. Ocular movements and vision appear to be normal in her right eye. She did not cooperate for fundoscopy.

Thinking pause.....
Isla is a young girl with a prosthetic left eye.

What may be the underlying diagnosis?
Isla may have been born with a congenital absence of her left eye but the eye socket appears to be normal and able to accommodate a prosthetic eye of comparable size to her other eye. The most likely diagnosis is that she has had retinoblastoma, requiring enucleation of her left eye and subsequent fitting of her prosthetic eye.

INTERNUCLEAR OPHTHALMOPLEGIA

STEM: This 10-year-old boy has difficulty looking to one side. Please examine his eyes.

PRESENTATION OF EXAMINATION FINDINGS

Andrew is a 10-year-old boy with abnormal eye movements. On lateral gaze to the left, the left eye abducts normally while the right eye fails to adduct. Lateral gaze to the right is normal. Visual field testing, pupillary reflexes and fundoscopy are all normal.

Thinking pause.....
Andrew has internuclear ophthalmoplegia.

Can you explain how lateral gaze is normally coordinated?

The medial longitudinal bundle connects the three ocular nerve nuclei to each other and to other nuclei, including the vestibular nuclei, coordinating the activity of the motor nerves to the eye. The parabducens nucleus, in the pons near to the abducens nucleus, coordinates conjugate lateral gaze. Fibres from here run to the VIth nucleus and to the contralateral IIIrd nerve nucleus via the medial longitudinal bundle. Voluntary gaze to the left is initiated in the right frontal cortex.

Can you explain this abnormality which is frequently poorly understood by candidates?

Internuclear ophthalmoplegia (INO) is due to a lesion within the median longitudinal fasciculus. In a right INO there is a lesion of the right median longitudinal fasciculus. On attempted left lateral gaze the right eye fails to adduct. The left eye develops coarse nystagmus in abduction. The site of the lesion is on the side of the impaired adduction, not the nystagmus. Destructive frontal lesions (e.g. tumour or infarct) cause failure of conjugate lateral gaze to the side opposite the lesion. In acute lesions the eyes are often deviated past the midline to the side of the lesion and therefore look *towards the normal limbs*. There is usually contralateral hemiparesis.

7 DEVELOPMENT

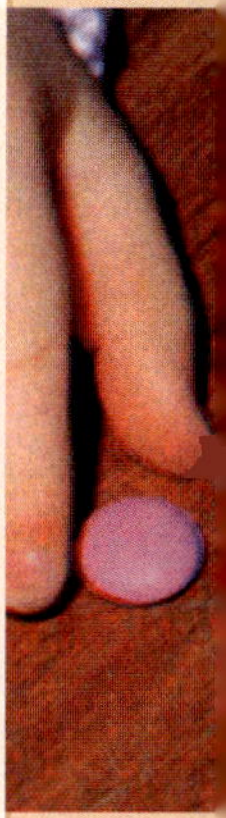

A GUIDE TO DEVELOPMENTAL ASSESSMENT

You may be asked to assess the development of a normal child in order to establish their age or, alternatively, the child may show delayed development for a given age. Remember that the normal range of development shows considerable variation between children. A summary of developmental milestones and developmental screening are presented in Tables 7.1 and 7.2 to help you determine a child's age or if development is appropriate. During the assessment of a child's development in the exam setting you may assess different milestones for the different categories in an unstructured manner depending on the cooperation of the child but try to present your findings in an organised fashion. For this reason it is often easier to present your findings as you progress with your assessment of development. Several examples are illustrated in the short cases below.

DEVELOPMENTAL ASSESSMENT SHORT CASES

DEVELOPMENTAL ASSESSMENT OF A 9-MONTH-OLD BOY

STEM: Please examine Matthew and tell me what age you think he is from your developmental assessment.

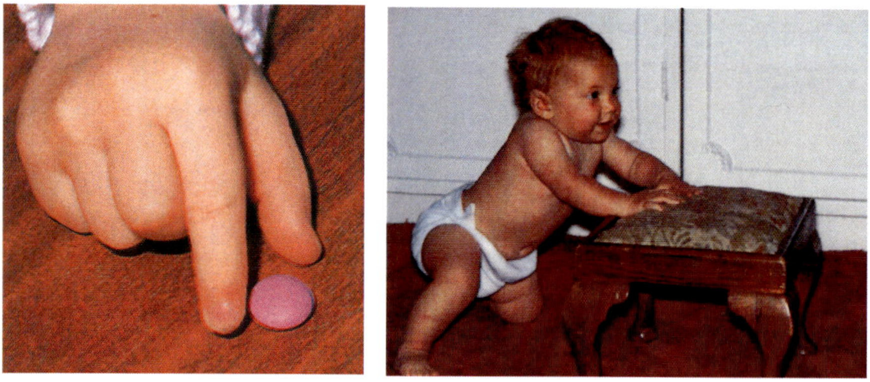

a b

Fig. 7.1 (**a**) *Pincer grip;* (**b**) *getting up to standing.*
(Reproduced with kind permission from Thomas R, Harvey D. Paediatrics: Colour Guide. Edinburgh: Churchill Livingstone, 1997.)

PRESENTATION OF EXAMINATION FINDINGS

Matthew sits alone and can lean forward to reach and pick up a toy without losing his balance. He is able to crawl on his knees, using his hands for support. He can pull himself to stand holding on to the furniture but is not yet able to stand alone, or cruise around the furniture. Matthew can reach out for small objects with a crude pincer grasp and he is able to point with his index finger. He releases toys on demand and looks for fallen objects. He can also roll a ball and pull a toy by the string. Matthew holds, bites and chews a biscuit but he is not yet able to drink from a cup or use a spoon. He also plays 'peek-a-boo' and understands several words. He does not appear to have any problems with his hearing and his parents have no concerns in this area, although I did not ask them if he passed his distraction hearing test.

Thinking pause.....
Matthew is an infant with the developmental age of a 9-month old boy.

DISSOCIATED DEVELOPMENTAL DELAY

STEM: Molly is a very active toddler but her parents are concerned that she says very little. Please assess her development and tell us what you find.

PRESENTATION OF EXAMINATION FINDINGS

Molly has a steady purposeful gait and is able to walk carrying a toy. She can run and squat. Molly can crawl up stairs and creeps downstairs. She enjoys books and points to the pictures and turns the pages. She is right handed and scribbles with a crayon. She can build a tower of three bricks. Molly helps to undress by taking off her socks and shoes. Molly drinks from a cup and feeds independently. She waves 'bye-bye' and looks for objects fallen out of sight. However, Molly does not appear to know her name or to respond to verbal commands. She has no speech and only very basic utterances. She does not turn to sound.

Thinking pause.....
Molly has the motor and social skills of an 18-month-old toddler but has no speech and does not appear to hear. She does not look like an ex-prem baby and has no dysmorphic features suggestive of an underlying syndrome. I would like to ask about her past medical history to establish whether she has any risk factors for deafness such as a history of meningitis, or family history of deafness. I would also like to know when the parents first became aware of a problem with Molly's hearing and what investigations have been performed.

Table 7.1 A guide to developmental assessment of the child in the exam setting

Age	Gross motor	Vision/fine motor	Hearing/speech	Personal/social
6 weeks	Symmetrical limb movements Ventral: head in line with body briefly Supine: fencing posture Automatic stepping and walking	Fixes and follows to 90° Turns to light Grasp reflex	Cries/coos Startles to noise	Smiles
3 months	Moves limbs vigorously No head lag Back: lumbar curvature only Prone: lifts upper chest up	Fixes and follows to 180° Plays with own hands Holds rattles placed in hand	Quietens to parent's voice Turns to sound	Laughs and squeals
6 months	Sits without support Lifts chest up on extended arms Grasps feet Rolls front to back Downward parachute	Palmar grasp Transfers objects Shakes rattle Mouths objects	Turns to quiet sound Says vowels and syllables	Laughs and screams Not shy
9 months	Tripod sits: rights self if pushed and can reach for toy steadily Rolls back to front Pulls to standing Stands holding on Forward parachute (7 months)	Reaches for small objects Rolls balls Points with index finger Early pincer grip Looks for fallen objects Releases toys	Distraction hearing test Says 'mama', 'dada', non-specifically	Chews biscuit Stranger anxiety Plays 'peek-a-boo' Understands 'no' and 'bye-bye'
12 months	Cruises around furniture Walks if held, may take a few steps unsupported	Neat pincer grip Casting objects Bangs cubes together	Knows name Understands simple commands Says a few words	Drinks from cup and uses spoon Finger-feeds Waves 'bye-bye' Finds hidden object

15 months	Broad-based gait Kneels Pushes wheeled toy	Sees small objects Tower of 2 bricks To and fro scribble	2–6 words Communicates wishes and obeys commands	Uses cup and spoon
18 months	Steady purposeful walk Runs, squats Walks carrying toy Pushes/pulls Creeps downstairs	Circular scribble Points to pictures in book Turns pages of book Hand preference	6–20 words	Points to named body parts Feeds independently Domestic mimicry Symbolic plays alone Takes off socks and shoes
2 years	Kicks ball Up and down stairs holding on	Tower of 6 bricks Copies vertical line	2–3 word sentences Uses pivotal grammar Uses question words	Feeds with fork and spoon Begins toilet training Temper tantrums
3 years	Up stairs 1 foot per step, down with 2 Walks on tip-toes Throws ball Pedals tricycle	Tower of 9 bricks Builds train and bridge with bricks if shown Copies circle	Gives first and last name Knows sex Recognises colours Pure tone audiometry	Washes hands and brushes teeth Eats with fork and spoon (± knife) Make-believe play Likes hearing and telling stories
4 years	Up and down stairs 1 foot per step Hops	Builds steps of bricks Copies cross Draws man	Counts to 10 or more	Able to undress
5 years	Skips Catches ball Runs on toes	Copies triangle	Asks ‘how’ and ‘when’ questions Uses grammatical speech	Uses knife and fork Able to put on clothes and to do large buttons

Table 7.2 Developmental screening

	Neonate	6 weeks	8–10 months	3–4 years	5 years
History	Pregnancy and delivery Any parental concerns	Birth details Illness to date Age of onset of: smiling, vocalization Response to sound Sucking and swallowing difficulties Risk factors for DDH: FH, breech, Caesarean section, talipes, torticollis, plagiocephaly Any parental concerns	Birth details As for 8–10 months plus age of onset of: holding rattle turning to sound reaching out and getting object sitting chewing crawling stand holding on (10 months) waves 'bye-bye' (10 months) Any words (10 months) Any parental concerns	Birth details As for 6 months plus age of onset of: walking alone joining words together extent of vocabulary speech understandable to strangers toilet trained ability to dress and feed himself Diet: iron deficiency peaks at 3 years Immunization history Any parental concerns	Any parental concerns: hearing vision, speech behaviour general health school Immunization history Any important life events

Examination	Measure and record: weight, length, OFC Observe alertness Dysmorphic features? Inspect: eyes for red reflex; mouth for cleft palate CVS/RS/GI/spine/feet Genitalia: testes descended hypospadias cliteromegaly Hips: developmental dislocation Barlow & Ortolani tests	Measure and record: weight, length, OFC Dysmorphic features Fontanelle Eyes: red reflex, squint, nystagmus CVS/RS/GI/genitalia Spine/hips Hold in ventral position Place prone Pull to sitting from supine Test weight bearing Test reflexes if tone or posture abnormal Test primitive reflexes (not essential)	Measure and record: weight, length, OFC Dysmorphic features Fontanelle Eyes: red reflex, squint, nystagmus CVS/RS/GI/genitalia Pull to sitting; sitting ability Observe grasp of raisin: test each eye finger–thumb apposition Test weight bearing Assess tone and reflexes if indicated Distraction hearing test Hips: assess for DDH by hip abduction	Measure and record: weight, height, OFC Dysmorphic features General physical exam Hip abduction Gait Standing on one leg/hop Manipulation of small objects Drawing a man Speech Test hearing and vision	Plot height and weight Visual acuity: Snellen chart Test hearing Examination: hair/skin/teeth/posture Interaction with parents

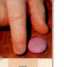

How would you assess hearing in a child of this age?

If there were concerns about Molly's hearing during the first 6 months of life she may have undergone a variety of tests including otoacoustic emission testing, which establishes if cochlear function is normal. Between 7 and 9 months of age all children undergo the distraction hearing test by trained professionals. Some children as young as 15 months of age may be able to cooperate with the speech discrimination test, although it is likely that Molly's hearing impairment was detected earlier.

Molly has a sensorineural loss. How would you manage this?

Molly should be looked after by a specialist team trained to assess the extent of her hearing impairment. Once this is established Molly will require early amplification with hearing aids for optimal speech and language development. Educational needs will require careful consideration and the multidisciplinary team will be involved in deciding whether Molly is able to attend a mainstream school with support or a school for children with severe hearing impairment. Intensive specialist teaching and support is provided by peripatetic teachers. Sensorineural hearing loss is irreversible and cochlear implants may be considered for Molly in the future.

8
SYNDROMES

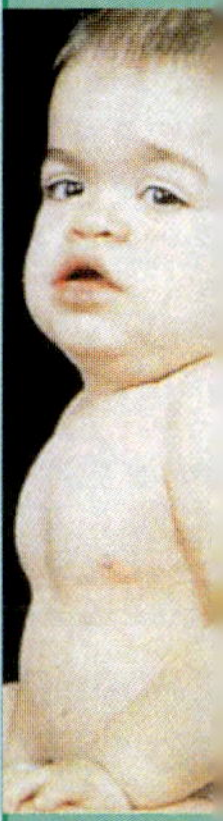

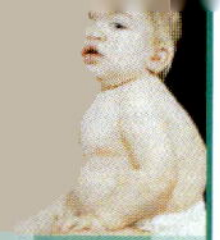

Often you will be asked to examine a child with a syndrome or condition you instantly recognise. Depending upon the request you may be able to give your answer in the form of a spot diagnosis. This will gain you full marks if you are correct but very little if you are wrong, so you must be certain of your diagnosis. More often you will be asked to examine the child and then formulate your diagnosis/differential diagnoses. If you do instantly recognise the condition then you have the advantage that you can actively look for the clinical features associated with that condition and can present your positive findings to support such a diagnosis. Below is a summary for examining a child with dysmorphic features. For a more detailed description we refer you to *Clinical Paediatrics for Postgraduate Examinations*, 3rd edition, by T Stephenson, H Wallace and A Thomson (Churchill Livingstone, Edinburgh, 2002).

SUMMARY FOR EXAMINING A CHILD WITH DYSMORPHIC FEATURES

INSPECTION

Head Does the size look normal and in proportion to the body? Micro/macrocephaly (maximum OFC: largest of 3, ask for centile chart). Is the shape normal? Are the sutures normal?

Eyes

- Is the face symmetrical? Do the eyes look abnormally close together or far apart? (e.g. Apert's, Crouzon's, Carpenter's)
- Know how to test for hypo/hypertelorism, microphthalmos, buphthalmos
- Epicanthic folds, palpebral fissures, synophrys, ptosis
- Orbital ridges: shallow or prominent?
- Corneal clouding, blue sclerae, heterochromia iridae, coloboma

Ears

- Low set? Know how to test for low-set ears
- Shape, size, auricular tags, accessory auricles
- Look with auriscope if necessary

Face

- Shape, symmetry, maxillary/mandibular hypoplasia
- Mouth: prominent lips; cleft lip or palate; gums hypertrophied, pigmented or ulcerated; high arched palate; macroglossia; tonsils; mouth ulcers; oral thrush
- Teeth: numbers, caries, pigmented
- Pallor, cyanosis

Hands Simian creases, brachydactyly, clinodactyly, polydactyly, syndactyly, arachnodactyly, broad thumbs, absent thumbs/radii

Skin Alopecia, hirsutism, pigmentation, depigmentation

Genitalia Cryptorchidism, hypospadias, micropenis

Once you have pieced together the dysmorphic features ask the examiner if you can now go on and examine the relevant system, e.g. cardiovascular system in Down's syndrome.

NEUROCUTANEOUS SYNDROMES

NEUROFIBROMATOSIS TYPE I

STEM: Olivia has attended the paediatric outpatient clinic regularly for review since she was noticed to have brown patches of skin by her GP a couple of years ago. Please examine her.

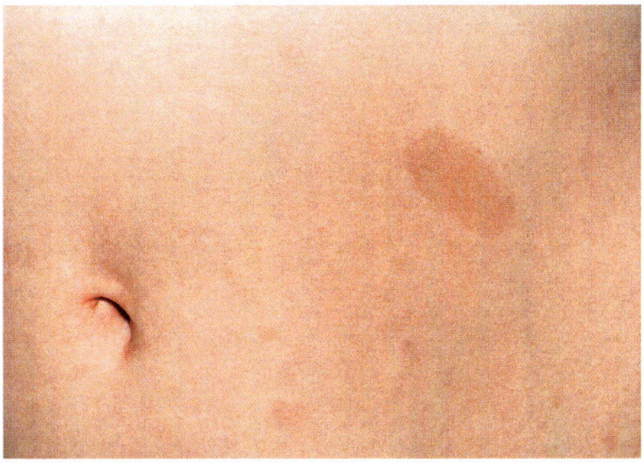

Fig. 8.1 *Café-au-lait patch seen in neurofibromatosis type I. Multiple patches of various sizes often occur.*

PRESENTATION OF EXAMINATION FINDINGS

Olivia is a teenage girl with multiple café-au-lait patches, each larger than 15 mm, and several neurofibromas on her abdomen. She also has axillary freckling. I could not see Lisch nodules and fundoscopy was normal. Olivia is a short girl with a relatively large head but I would like to confirm these observations by plotting her height, weight and head circumference on a growth chart appropriate for her age and sex. She has no evidence of scoliosis and her blood pressure is within the normal range. Her mother is with her and she also has café-au-lait patches and neurofibromas.

Thinking pause.....
In summary, this is a well girl with neurofibromatosis type I.

What can you tell me about neurofibromatosis?
This is the most common of the neurocutaneous syndromes. There are eight types described of which type I accounts for 90% of cases. Neurofibromatosis type I has an incidence of 1 in 4000. It is inherited autosomal dominantly with the gene locus mapped to chromosome 17,

although 50% of cases are new mutations. Diagnosis is made by fulfilling two of the following criteria:

1. Six or more café au lait macules: >5 mm = prepubertal; >15 mm = post pubertal
2. Two or more neurofibromas or one plexiform neurofibroma
3. Axillary or inguinal freckling
4. Optic glioma (15%)
5. Two or more Lisch nodules (iris hamartomas)
6. Family history

What are the associated features and complications?

- Macrocephaly (46% >97th centile)
- Short stature (34% <3rd centile)
- Mild learning difficulties (30%)
- Scoliosis (11.5%)
- Hypertension: renal artery stenosis (2%), phaeochromocytoma (3%)
- Malignancy: optic glioma, astrocytoma, schwannoma, rhabdomyosarcoma
- Seizures
- Osseous lesions, e.g. kyphoscoliosis, tibial bowing, pseudoarthrosis

What other causes of café-au-lait spots do you know?

- Ataxic telangiectasia
- Tuberous sclerosis
- Fanconi's anaemia
- McCune–Albright syndrome
- Russell–Silver dwarfism
- Bloom's syndrome
- Gaucher's disease
- Chediak–Higashi syndrome
- Normal variant

TUBEROUS SCLEROSIS

STEM: Kirsty first presented to the paediatric department when she was 8 months old with a history of afebrile seizures, and has been reviewed regularly. Please examine her.

PRESENTATION OF EXAMINATION FINDINGS

Kirsty is a girl with adenoma sebaceum, ashleaf spots on her forearms and trunk and a few shagreen patches above her sacrum. Her development appears to be delayed. She usually wears a protective helmet and I would presume that she continues to have seizures.

Thinking pause.....
This is a girl with tuberous sclerosis.

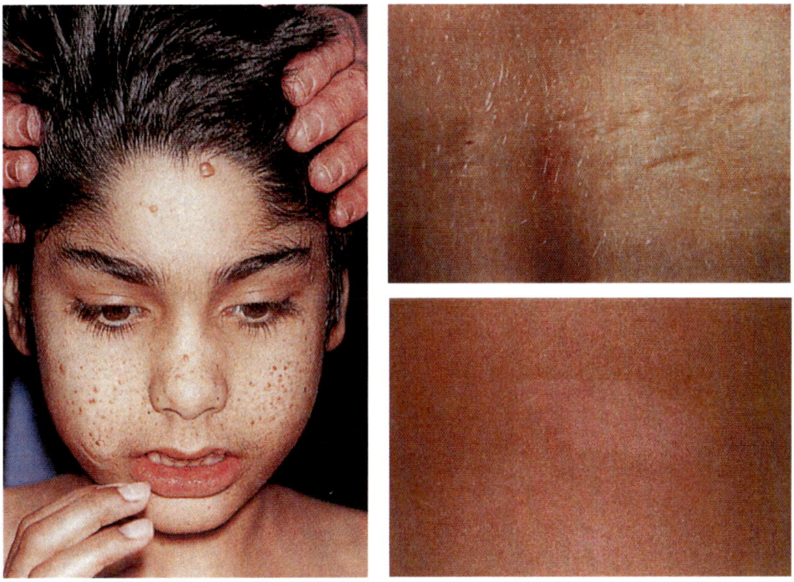

Fig. 8.2 *Tuberous sclerosis:* (**a**) *adenoma sebaceum;* (**b**) *Shagreen patch;* (**c**) *depigmented patches.*
(Reproduced with kind permission from McIntosh N, Helms P J, Smyth R L (eds) Forfar & Arneil's Textbook of Pediatrics, 6th edn. Edinburgh: Churchill Livingstone, 2003.)

What can you tell me about this condition?

This is a neurocutaneous syndrome commonly associated with epilepsy and intellectual impairment. It shows an autosomal dominant inheritance, although 70% are new mutations, and an incidence of 1 in 10 000 to 50 000. The gene for tuberous sclerosis is on the long arm of chromosome 9, named TSCI. A second tuberous sclerosis locus has been identified on the proximal side of the polycystic kidney disease type I (PKDI) gene on chromosome 16p13, which has been designated TSC2 and appears to be a tumour suppressor gene.

Seizures are common and often present as infantile spasms and are difficult to control. The age of onset of seizures and degree of intellectual impairment are directly related. Other clinical features are shown in Box 8.1 (see next page).

STURGE–WEBER SYNDROME

STEM: Sam is a 7-year-old boy who is under the care of the community paediatrician and attends a school for children with special needs. Please examine him.

PRESENTATION OF EXAMINATION FINDINGS

Sam is a young boy with a facial port wine stain in the distribution of the trigeminal nerve with particular emphasis over the ophthalmic area. He appears to have a mild contralateral hemiplegia. Although he looks about

Box 8.1 Clinical features of tuberous sclerosis

Skin
- Adenoma sebaceum (present in 85% of children >5 years old)
- Ashleaf spots (hypopigmented macules)
- Shagreen patches
- Periungual fibromas (onset at puberty)
- Café-au-lait patches occasionally

Eyes
- Retinal phakomata (40%)

Teeth
- Enamel hypoplasia

CNS
- Tuberous hamartomata (in 90% may calcify)
- Seizures (any type)
- Cerebral astrocytoma, malignant glioma, hydrocephalus
- Intellectual impairment (40%), all have seizures; if normal intellect, seizure rate is about 60%.

CVS
Rhabdomyoma

Renal
- Polycystic kidney disease (chromosome 16)
- Renal angiomas

Gastrointestinal
- Rectal polyp

7 years old his development appears to be considerably delayed just upon observation of his play.

Thinking pause.....
Sam is a young boy with Sturge–Weber syndrome.

Anything else?
I would like to ask his parents if he suffers from epilepsy.

What is a port wine stain?
It is a cavernous haemangioma, which in Sturge–Weber syndrome affects one or more areas of the trigeminal nerve, particularly the ophthalmic division, associated with a haemangiomatous lesion of the brain. This can be seen as intracranial calcification on skull X-ray, or more clearly on CT scan. It is present from birth and is associated with epilepsy, contralateral hemiplegia and mental retardation in 30%. Children presenting with intractable epilepsy in early infancy may benefit from hemispherectomy.

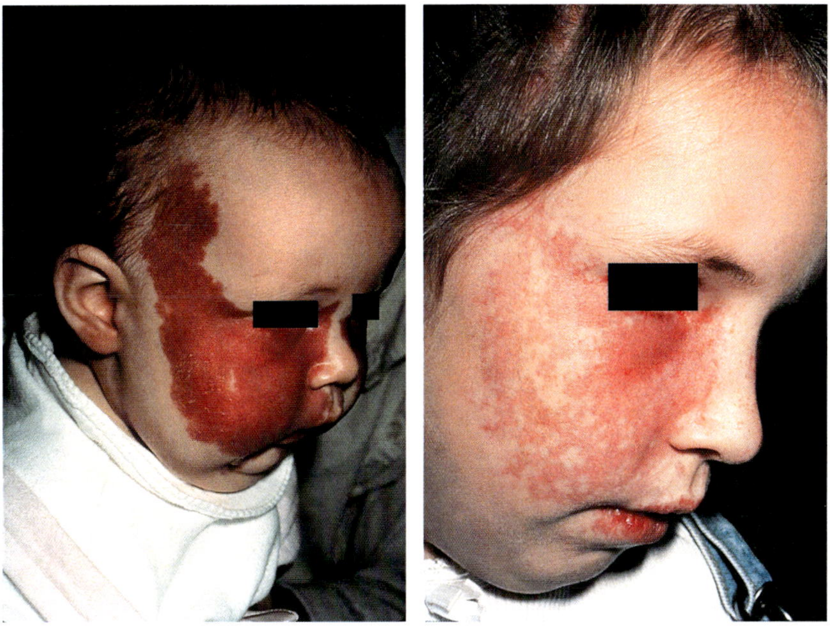

a b

Fig. 8.3 *Port wine stain V2 dermatome.* (**a**) *Before laser treatment;* (**b**) *after eight laser treatments the lesion is considerably lighter but still persists.*
(Reproduced with kind permission from Schachner L A, Hansen R C. Pediatric Dermatology, 3rd edn. Edinburgh: Mosby, 2003.)

Can anything be done to improve the cosmetic appearance of the port wine stain?

Laser treatment of the port wine stain can be commenced once the seizures are controlled by anticonvulsants.

What other causes do you know of intracranial calcification?

- Tuberous sclerosis
- Arteriovenous malformations
- Congenital infections – toxoplasmosis, CMV, rubella
- Brain tumours – glioma, astrocytoma, craniopharyngioma

NEURODEGENERATIVE DISORDERS

HURLER'S SYNDROME

> **STEM:** Greig is an 18-month-old boy who was referred to the paediatric department by his GP at age 8 months following concerns that he had some facial dysmorphism and was developing slowly. Please examine him.

PRESENTATION OF EXAMINATION FINDINGS

Greig is a young boy with a coarse face with thickened skin and a large tongue with thick lips. He has hypertrichosis, especially on his face, and

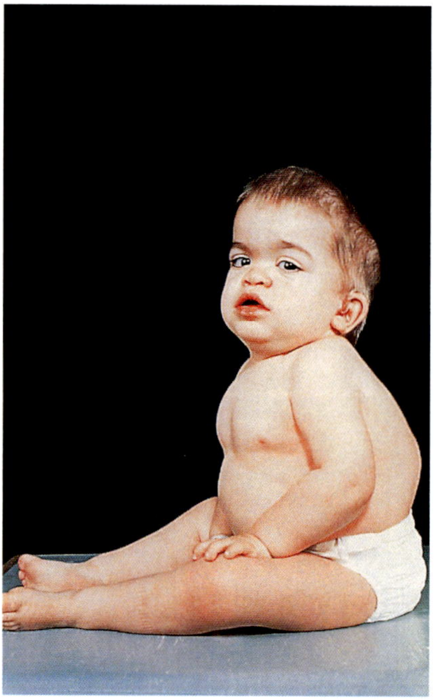

Fig. 8.4 *Hurler's syndrome showing the characteristic facies and skeletal dysplasia.* (Reproduced with kind permission from Lissauer T, Clayden G. Illustrated Textbook of Paediatrics, 2nd edn. Edinburgh: Mosby, 2001.)

frontal bossing. The red reflex is absent in keeping with corneal clouding. When sitting on his parent's knee, he clearly has a thoracolumbar kyphosis and a lumbar lordosis. He has broad claw hands. Greig appears to be of short stature although ideally I would like to plot his height and weight on a growth chart appropriate for his age and sex.

On examination of the cardiovascular system he has an ejection systolic murmur loudest over the upper left sternal edge in keeping with pulmonary outflow tract obstruction. Palpation of his abdomen revealed hepatosplenomegaly.

Thinking pause.....
In summary this is a young boy with Hurler's syndrome.

What is Hurler's syndrome?

This is type I of the mucopolysaccharide storage disorders of which there are seven different types. It is of autosomal recessive inheritance. The mucopolysaccharidoses are progressive multisystem disorders which may affect any system, particularly the neurological, ocular, cardiac and skeletal systems. As with the other neurodegenerative disorders the cardinal feature at presentation is developmental regression, in this case following a period of normal growth and development up until 6–12 months of age. From about age 6 months onwards these children develop coarsened features with the characteristic facial appearance.

How is this condition diagnosed?

It is a disorder of the major storage substance, glycosaminoglycans, due to a defect of the enzyme, α-L-iduronidase, which is coded for on chromosome 22. Identification of the enzyme defect and increased secretion of dermatan and heparin sulphate in the urine is the key to diagnosis. These infants also require ophthalmology, cardiology and neurological assessment to look for associated problems.

What is the prognosis for such children?

Unfortunately the prognosis is poor and treatment is supportive to the children's needs. Ear and chest infections and cardiac failure are common. Glaucoma should be anticipated and treated early. Decompression may be required for carpal tunnel syndrome. Occupational therapy and physiotherapy may be helpful. Adequate support for the family is also essential. Generally these children die from cardiovascular or respiratory disease in the first decade. Enzyme replacement by bone marrow transplant has been performed in a few of the most severe cases with some improvement.

HUNTER'S SYNDROME

STEM: Simon is 5-year-old boy who first presented to his GP at 2 years of age because his parents were concerned that he was developing a hump. Please examine him.

PRESENTATION OF EXAMINATION FINDINGS

Simon is a young boy with coarse facies and frontal bossing. He has a large tongue and thick lips. He is of short stature with moderate kyphoscoliosis and clawed hands. His red reflexes are intact. Over his scapular area he has skin nodules. Cardiovascular examination appeared to be normal and on abdominal palpation he had mild hepatosplenomegaly.

Thinking pause.....

This is a young boy with Hunter's syndrome.

Why do you say Hunter's syndrome?

Although it is very similar to Hurler's syndrome he does not appear to have corneal involvement and the skin nodules on the scapulae are characteristic of Hunter's syndrome. Hunter's syndrome is X-linked unlike all the other mucopolysaccharidoses. It is also associated with cardiomyopathy and this boy should have a cardiac ultrasound scan. Hunter's syndrome also tends to run a more benign course than Hurler's syndrome.

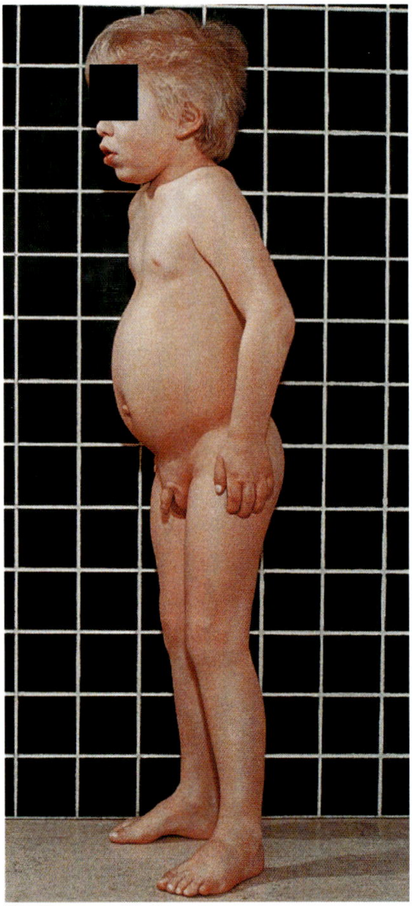

Fig. 8.5 *Mucopolysaccharidosis II emphasising the relatively long legs compared with back.*
(Reproduced with kind permission from Wales J K H, Wit J-M, Rogol A D. Pediatric Endocrinology and Growth, 2nd edn. Edinburgh: Saunders, 2003.)

LYSOSOMAL STORAGE DISORDERS: GAUCHER'S DISEASE (pronounced Goshey's disease)

> **STEM:** Emily is a 7-year-old girl who was found to have an incidental radiological abnormality when she presented to the Accident and Emergency Department following an injury to her leg after she fell off her bike. As there were no fractures to her lower limbs Emily was discharged home. You were contacted by the radiologist and prompted to contact the family to bring Emily for further assessment. Please examine her.

PRESENTATION OF EXAMINATION FINDINGS

Emily is a well nourished girl with no dysmorphic features. She has a few patches of yellow–brown skin pigmentation on her trunk. The only other abnormal finding is moderate splenomegaly. I would like to know if she has a history of bone pain, other than the recent trauma, or fractures and any haematological complications due to hypersplenism.

Thinking pause.....

This is a young girl with a large spleen, with yellow–brown skin pigmentation who is otherwise well. The underlying diagnosis may be Gaucher's disease. I would like to see her X-rays as I would suspect that the X-ray abnormality may show the classical Erlenmeyer flask deformity.

What is Gaucher's disease?

This autosomal recessive disease is the commonest of the lysosomal storage disorders and is due to a deficiency of glucosylceramide β-glucosidase activity resulting in accumulation of glucosylceramide. Three types of Gaucher's disease exist: chronic Type I, acute Type II and subacute Type III. Type I is the most prevalent form, common among Ashkenazi Jews, and presents with hepatosplenomegaly during childhood or young adulthood. Haematological complications may occur due to hypersplenism and this can be partly relieved by splenectomy. More recently, replacement treatment has been available. Bony infiltration also occurs causing pain and patchy osteopenia and osteonecrosis leading to fractures and considerable disability. Expansion of the cortex of the distal femur produces the characteristic X-ray appearances known as Erlenmeyer flask deformity.

Acute neuropathic Type II presents in early infancy with hepatosplenomegaly and marked neurological complications of brainstem involvement. Death is usually due to gross failure to thrive secondary to feeding and breathing problems within the first 2 years of life. Subacute neuropathic Type III is a severe form of Type I and may be associated with seizures, with variable prognosis.

How would you confirm the diagnosis?

Demonstration of deficient β-glucosidase activity in leucocytes or fibroblasts is diagnostic in all three types.

DOWN'S SYNDROME

STEM: Jeremy is a 6-year-old boy who attends a school for children with special needs and is under regular review by the community paediatrician. Please examine him.

PRESENTATION OF EXAMINATION FINDINGS

Jeremy is a short 6-year-old boy with a round face with a flat occiput. He has epicanthic folds, upward-sloping palpebral fissures and Brushfield spots. He has a flat nasal bridge and a protruding tongue due to a relatively small

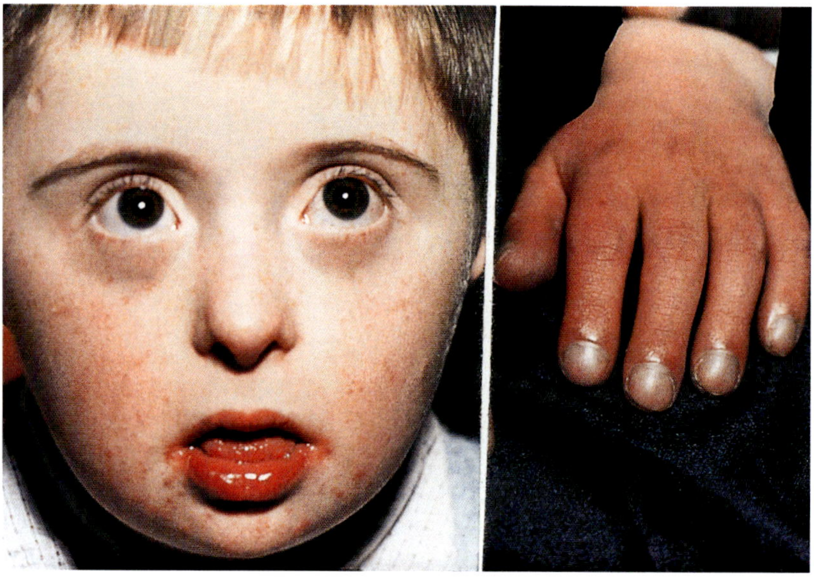

a

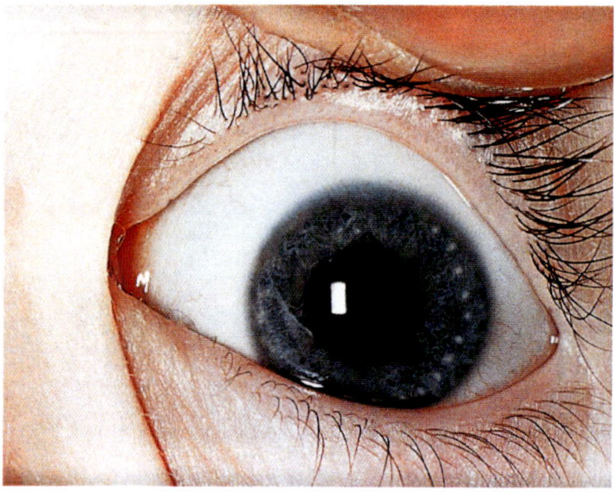

b

Fig. 8.6 (**a**) *Typical facial appearance of Down's syndrome. Cyanosis and clubbed fingers indicate cyanotic heart disease, a recognised finding in this syndrome.* (**b**) *The speckled appearance of the iris – 'Brushfield spots'.*
(Reproduced with kind permission from TALC. Image©Teaching-aids At Low Cost)

mouth. His ears are small with an overfolding helix and his hair is fine and sparse. Jeremy has small broad hands with clinodactyly of the fifth fingers and abnormal dermatoglyphics. His posture is due to hypotonia. He has a wide 'sandal' gap between his first and second toes and also a deep plantar crease. I would like to plot his height and weight on a growth chart for a male child with Down's syndrome.

Thinking pause.....

Jeremy is a boy with the characteristic phenotype of a child with Down's syndrome.

What do you mean by abnormal dermatoglyphics?

Jeremy has bilateral single palmar or simian creases. He also has an increase in ulnar loops, a single flexion crease of his fifth fingers and a distal axial triradius.

What other systems would you like to examine?

It is important to examine the cardiovascular system as congenital heart disease occurs in 40–60% of these children, most commonly atrioventricular canal defects. I would like to examine his eyes to exclude cataracts and squints. Examination of his ears to look for secretory otitis media and assessment of hearing are also important.

Can you explain the cytogenetics of Down's syndrome?

Approximately 95% of cases are due to trisomy 21 as result of meiotic non-disjunction usually from the maternal side and the incidence rises with increasing maternal age. Translocation occurs in 3–4% with translocation of a chromosome 21 onto chromosome 14, or more rarely to 15, 22 or 21, known as a Robertsonian translocation. In about a quarter of these children the parent carries a balanced translocation with the risk of recurrence higher if the mother is the carrier, at about 10–15%. If the translocation in either parent is 21:21, all the offspring will have Down's syndrome. Mosaicism accounts for the remainder, usually due to non-disjunction at mitosis.

What other problems are associated with Down's syndrome?

These children have a higher incidence of intestinal atresia, especially duodenal atresia, accounting for one-third of all cases of congenital duodenal atresia. Developmental milestones are delayed due to hypotonia and a varying degree of learning difficulties with IQ ranging from 20 to 75.

Puberty delay is usual in both sexes with normal female fertility and universal male infertility. Hypothyroidism is common and routine screening is essential. The incidence of leukaemia is 10–18 times greater than that of the general population with AML commoner in early life and ALL predominating in older children. Presenile dementia is common in adulthood.

What is the relationship between Down's syndrome and Alzheimer's disease?

The neuropathology is similar in both conditions with senile plaques and neurofibrillary tangles. However, in Down's syndrome there is a generalised depletion of all neurotransmitters, whereas in Alzheimer's there is a depletion of cholinergic neurotransmitters. Interestingly, a predisposing gene locus has been identified on chromosome 21 in some familial cases with early onset Alzheimer's.

TURNER'S SYNDROME

STEM: Amy is an 11-year-old girl who regularly attends the endocrine clinic. Please examine her.

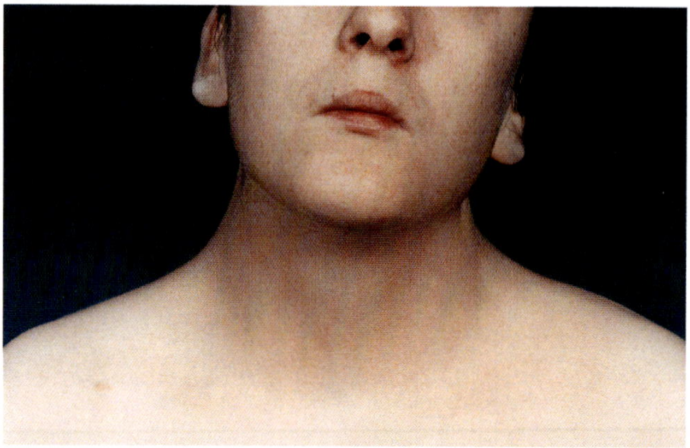

a

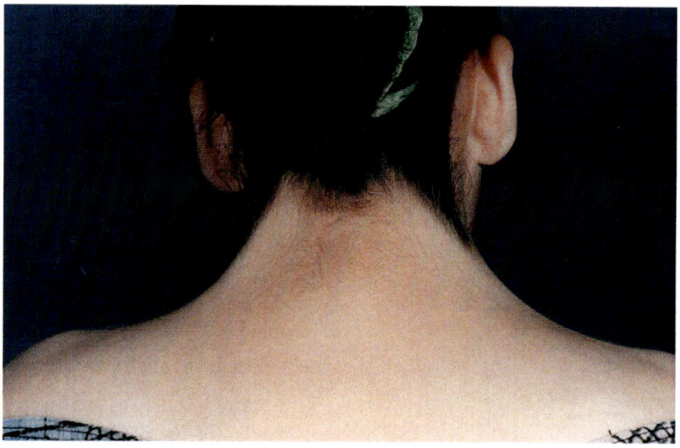

b

Fig. 8.7 (**a, b**) *A girl with Turner's syndrome showing webbing of the neck.*

PRESENTATION OF EXAMINATION FINDINGS

Amy is an 11-year-old girl who is of short stature and has webbing of the neck with a low posterior hairline. Her eyes show soft dysmorphism of the palpebral fissures and she has mildly dysplastic ears. She has a high pointed arched palate, known as a Gothic palate, giving her voice a nasal quality. She has widely spaced nipples, increased pigmented naevi and increased body hair, especially on the extensor surfaces of her lower arms. When her arms are completely extended there is cubitus valgus or a wide carrying angle. Her toenails and fingernails are concave. She has short fingers with a particularly short fourth metacarpal and similarly the fourth toes are also short.

Thinking pause.....

Amy has the characteristic phenotype of Turner's syndrome. I would like to ask about her birth weight and if there was any puffiness of the hands and feet. I would also like to know whether Amy had any feeding difficulties during the neonatal period.

Anything else?

I would like to examine her cardiovascular system as these children have an increased incidence of congenital heart disease. The most common abnormality is stenosis of the aortic isthmus, coarctation at the beginning of the descending aorta, which is corrected surgically. Other cardiac abnormalities include bicuspid aortic valve, aortic stenosis and aortic aneurysms.

Monitoring of growth and pubertal development is essential, as these children have short stature and failure of puberty. I would like to plot her height and weight on a Turner's syndrome growth chart.

How is growth failure managed in these children?

Body length at birth is below the norm and, with slower growth velocity, their height deviates further from the norm with progressive age. The mean final height lies between 142 and 147 cm ± 12 cm. There are two options for the management of growth failure:

- *Steroid treatment* – oxandrolone, an anabolic steroid with minimal androgenic side effects, if used in low doses will increase final adult height.
- *Growth hormone* – recombinant growth hormone alone, or in combination with oxandrolone, increases final height by about 6–8 cm. Higher doses are required in Turner's syndrome than in growth hormone deficiency.

There is no evidence to support the use of oestrogens to increase adult height. Oestrogens accelerate the closure of the epiphyseal cartilage and the development of normal physical characteristics may be at the expense of an early end to growth.

What are her prospects for fertility?

Ovarian dysgenesis results in infertility in the majority of patients. The ovary develops normally until 14–16 weeks' gestation and then oocytes are lost and replaced with connective tissue. Consequently there is failure of puberty due to hypergonadotrophic hypogonadism, although about 10% of girls retain sufficient ovarian function for puberty to commence. In a few cases spontaneous menarche occurs and there have also been a few reports of spontaneous pregnancies. The majority of children require oestrogen replacement at the age of 12–13 years for the development of normal secondary sexual characteristics. With advances in assisted reproductive techniques, pregnancy can be achieved in these patients. The structure of the uterus, vagina and external genitalia is normal and pregnancy with in vitro fertilisation of a donor oocyte is possible.

Renal abnormalities are also common and include 'horseshoe kidney', malposition, duplicate renal pelvis and ureters, increase in number of renal vessels or abnormal vessel course. These can be detected on ultrasound scan but most of the changes are of no consequence to renal function.

A summary of the characteristic features of Turner's syndrome is shown in Table 8.1. The features of Noonan's syndrome are included for comparison.

Table 8.1 Characteristic features of Turner's and Noonan's syndromes

	Turner	Noonan
Sex	Female Not inherited 45XO (50%), 50% partial X or isochromosome X	Male or female Usually sporadic Autosomal dominance with variable penetrance occurs Gene defect – chromosome 12
Phenotype	Short stature Delayed puberty Webbing of the neck Cubitus valgus Shield chest High arched palate Anti-mongoloid slant Ptosis Micrognathia	Short stature (50%) Delayed puberty Webbing of the neck Cubitus valgus Shield chest High arched palate Anti-mongoloid slant Ptosis Micrognathia
Birth	Short at birth Feeding difficulties Lymphoedema of hands and feet	Normal length Feeding difficulties
Cardiac defects	Coarctation of aorta	Pulmonary stenosis
Mental abilities	Usually normal	Impaired in 40%
Gonads/fertility	Ovarian dysgenesis Most are infertile	Normal gonads Most are fertile
Other features	Renal abnormalities Thyroid disorders increased	Bleeding disorders

FRAGILE X SYNDROME

STEM: Callum requires a lot of extra support at school and the school doctor wondered if he was dysmorphic and requested a second opinion. Please examine him.

PRESENTATION OF EXAMINATION FINDINGS

Callum is a 6-year-old boy with soft dysmorphic facial features. He has a large head with a large forehead and long prominent ears. His nose is long and his chin prominent. Callum has soft skin and joint hypermobility. His intelligence is moderately reduced, although not formally assessed. I would like to plot his height and weight on a growth chart appropriate for his age and sex and to assess his pubertal status.

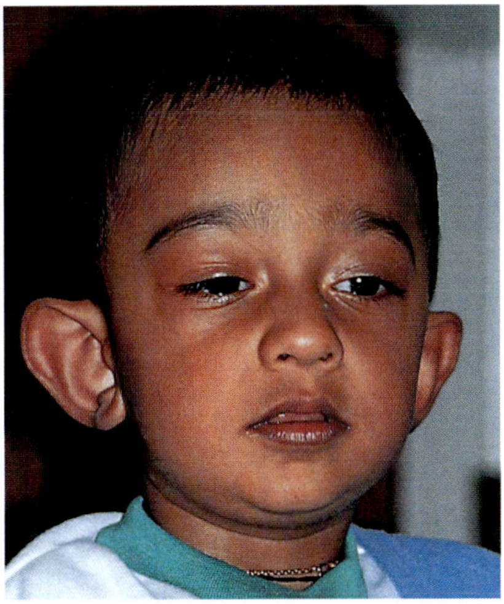

Fig. 8.8 *A child with fragile X syndrome. At this age, the main feature is often the prominent ears.*
(Reproduced with kind permission from Lissauer T, Clayden G. Illustrated Textbook of Paediatrics, 2nd edn. Edinburgh: Mosby, 2001.)

Thinking pause.....
Callum is a young boy with a phenotype in keeping with fragile X syndrome. Assessment of pubertal status is likely to reveal macro-orchidism.

How is this condition diagnosed?

Fragile X is the second most common genetic cause of severe learning difficulties after Down's syndrome. It is inherited as a sex linked recessive disorder but expression is due to the process of allelic expansion. The fragile site is on the long arm of chromosome X at Xq27.3, which gives the appearance of an isochromatid gap.

What about fragile X in females?

About one-third of female heterozygotes may show some manifestations of the syndrome, usually in the form of mild developmental delay but it can be severe. The transmission causes an increase in the fragile repeats and there appears to be some correlation between the level of expression of fragile sites and the reduction in intelligence.

RUBINSTEIN–TAYBI SYNDROME

STEM: Thomas was noticed to have funny thumbs by his parents when he was a toddler. Please examine him.

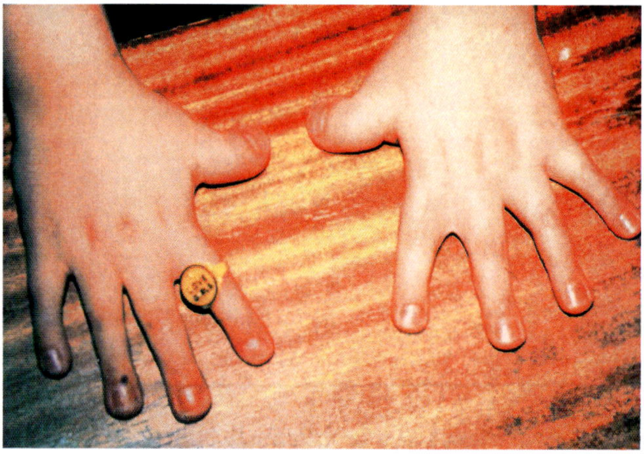

Fig. 8.9 *A boy with Rubenstein–Taybi syndrome showing broad thumbs which are radially angled. He also has webbing of his fingers.*

PRESENTATION OF EXAMINATION FINDINGS

Thomas is a 7-year-old boy with soft dysmorphic facial features. He has a small head with a beaked nose, prominent columella. He has polydactyly and his thumbs are abnormally broad bilaterally. His toes are also short, broad and webbed. His play and speech are immature for his age, suggesting that he has learning difficulties, although I have not formally assessed his development. I would also like to plot his height and weight on a growth chart appropriate for his age and sex.

Thinking pause.....
Thomas is a boy with features in keeping with a diagnosis of Rubinstein–Taybi syndrome.

How would you confirm the diagnosis?
Genetic tests are available to assist with the diagnosis. Rubinstein–Taybi is associated with a microdeletion of chromosome 16p13 and may be detected in 20% of cases using FISH studies.

What is the differential diagnosis of a broad thumb?
Other syndromes associated with a broad thumb include Apert's, Carpenter's and Larsen syndromes.

RUSSELL–SILVER SYNDROME

STEM: Gillian is a 15-month-old girl, born at term by SVD, following a normal pregnancy and weighed 2.3 kg. Her GP referred her to the paediatric clinic following concerns by the health visitor that she was short. Please examine her.

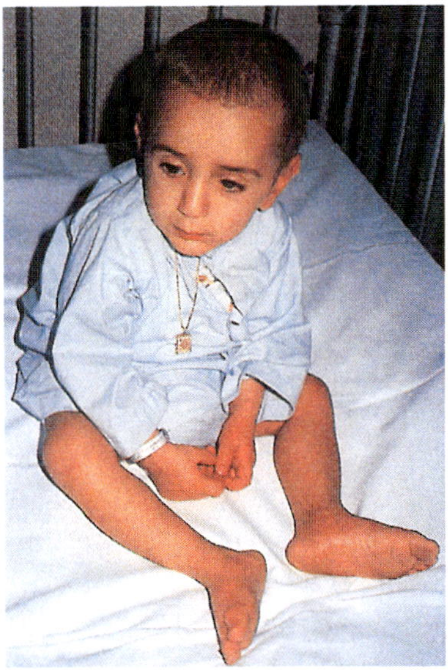

Fig. 8.10 *Russell–Silver syndrome: note the small triangular facies.*
(Reproduced with kind permission from Thomas R, Harvey D. Paediatrics: Colour Guide. Edinburgh: Churchill Livingstone, 1997.)

PRESENTATION OF EXAMINATION FINDINGS

Gillian is a small 15-month-old girl with dysmorphic facies. Her face is small and triangular with frontal bossing and prominent ears. Her lips are thin and she has micrognathia. She has mild limb asymmetry and clinodactyly of the fifth finger. I also note that she has a few café-au-lait patches. Her play and speech are appropriate for her age. I would like to plot her head circumference, height and weight on a growth chart appropriate for her age and sex, to confirm that she has short stature.

Thinking pause.....
This little girl has the characteristic appearance of Russell–Silver syndrome.

What is this condition?
This is a chromosomal disorder associated with short stature and characteristic facies. The children are usually born with intrauterine growth retardation. Development is usually normal and the characteristic phenotype disappears with increasing age.

Box 8.2 Characteristics of Russell–Silver syndrome

Almost without exception, sufferers of RSS have the following traits:

- Low birth weight (IUGR)
- Decreased birth length
- Triangular-shaped facies (lessens with age)
- Scaphocephaly (long narrow head) at birth
- Apparent neonatal large head due to relative short body length and low birth weight
- Poor feeding in early years
- Clinodactyly of fifth finger

Common characteristics

- Hypoglycaemia in infancy and early childhood (first 2–3 years)
- Asymmetry (side-to-side, one side larger than the other)
- Delayed closure of fontanelle
- Broad forehead
- Micrognathia
- Downturned corners of the mouth
- Thin upper lip
- Crowding of teeth and microdontia
- High-pitched voice (usually disappears in later life)
- Low-set ears and/or prominent ears
- Syndactyly of toes
- Hypospadias
- Cryptorchidism
- Delayed bone age
- Weak muscle tone
- Learning difficulties

Rarer features

- Hydrocephalus
- Blue sclerae
- High arched palate
- Congenital absence of second premolars
- Café-au-lait patches
- Frequent ear infection or chronic glue ear
- Vertebral anomalies
- Renal anomalies
- Scoliosis
- Reflux
- Migraines
- Growth hormone deficiency
- Precocious puberty
- High energy/ADHD
- Reflex anoxic syncope

How is this condition inherited?

Genetic problems are thought to cause this syndrome, although the specific gene(s) remain to be discovered. The pattern of inheritance has not been determined, but in most cases it seems to occur without any family history of the condition.

One interesting aspect of this condition is the wide variation of clinical characteristics associated with it. Some subjects have many of the traits whereas others have only a few (Box 8.2). Mental retardation is not characteristic of this disorder.

How are these children managed?

Management of these children is generally multidisciplinary to ensure all the child's needs are met:

- These children are referred to a geneticist initially to confirm the diagnosis, and to an endocrinologist to determine which physical anomalies might need treatment
- Dietary support – may be necessary to avoid hypoglycaemia spells. Most children will require nutritional support as poor appetite is common. Some children may require gastrostomy feeding to provide adequate calorie intake
- Growth hormone may be appropriate to increase final height, particularly where GHD has been shown
- Speech therapy
- Physiotherapy
- Occupational therapy
- Grommet insertion
- Limb lengthening surgery

What is the long-term outcome for these children?

Children with RSS do not necessarily have a reduced quality of life. Many of the traits improve with time. The phenotype becomes less pronounced, muscle tone and motor coordination improve. Appetite increases and speech improves. Short stature tends to be a persistent feature and most adults will be less than 5 feet tall, although this is improving for children who respond to growth hormone replacement therapy. Most children live a normal life and become healthy adults.

DiGEORGE'S SYNDROME (Velo-cardio-facial or Shprintzen syndrome)

STEM: Elizabeth is a 3-year-old girl who presented with seizures in the neonatal period. Please examine her.

PRESENTATION OF EXAMINATION FINDINGS

Elizabeth is a young girl with low-set, abnormally formed ears, hypertelorism and downward-sloping palpebral fissures. She has a prominent nose, micrognathia, a short philtrum to the upper lip and a high arched palate. She is pink and well perfused in air with no finger clubbing. She has long elegant fingers. Elizabeth has a right thoracotomy scar and midline sternotomy scar. Her speech is somewhat nasal in quality and she has previously had a cleft lip repaired. She is a small slight girl with reduced subcutaneous tissues and I would like to plot her on a growth chart appropriate for her age and sex.

Thinking pause.....

Elizabeth has the phenotype and evidence of corrective surgery for congenital cardiac disease in keeping with a diagnosis of DiGeorge's syndrome.

What is DiGeorge's syndrome?

This syndrome is a rare type of immunodeficiency syndrome with an incidence of about 1 in 66 000. It results from abnormal embryological development of the third and fourth pharyngeal arch structures. In the full-blown syndrome there is immunodeficiency and hypocalcaemia secondary to hypoparathyroidism. A variety of congenital heart defects have been reported to result from interruption of the branchial arch, including tetralogy of Fallot, pulmonary artery and aorta anomalies.

How is this condition inherited?

It usually occurs sporadically, associated with a chromosome 22q deletion, although it can be dominantly inherited with subtle features in the parents. Parents must therefore be tested because this would lead to a 50% risk of disease in further progeny. Confirmation of cytogenetic abnormality can be made by FISH studies.

What can you tell me about the associated immunodeficiency?

The immune deficiency is a consequence of absent thymus and is primarily a cell-mediated deficiency. This means the children are excessively prone to candidiasis, recurrent pneumonias (typical and atypical), diarrhoea and failure to thrive.

How would you test cell-mediated immunity?

In DiGeorge's syndrome there will be a T-cell deficiency. In the normal healthy individual, T-cells constitute around two-thirds of the circulating lymphocytes, so T-cell numbers can be estimated using a number of techniques such as monoclonal antibody tests or erythrocyte rosetting. Alternatively, lymphocyte function may be tested by demonstrating poor mitogen responses, antigenic responses and cytotoxic function. These patients may also develop hypogammaglobulinaemia.

What is the prognosis for this condition?

The syndrome is extremely heterogeneous and partial forms are more common than the full-blown condition. Occasionally, in the less severe types, spontaneous improvement in immune function may occur. Treatment of the immune deficiency has been successfully achieved using fetal thymus implants or bone marrow transplants, and some success with thymic hormones or cultured thymic epithelial implants has been reported. The main determinants in the full-blown condition are cardiac and metabolic problems.

PRADER–WILLI SYNDROME

STEM: Dylan is a 5-year-old boy who was referred to the paediatric clinic by his GP following concerns that he was overeating and consequently gaining weight rapidly despite input from the dietician. Please examine him.

PRESENTATION OF EXAMINATION FINDINGS

Dylan is an overweight boy who appears to be of short stature. He has a narrow forehead and fair hair. He has upward-sloping palpebral fissures and almond-shaped blue eyes with strabismus. He has mild micrognathia and a thin upper lip. Dylan has small hands and feet with clinodactyly of the fifth fingers bilaterally. His tone is diminished and his development appears to be delayed. On examination of his abdomen I note that he has hypogonadism with micropenis.

Thinking pause.....
This is a boy with Prader–Willi syndrome.

Would you like to ask his parents any questions?

- 'Did the doctors comment on Dylan being quite floppy as a baby?'
- 'Did Dylan have any feeding problems as a baby?'

I would also like to ask about Dylan's educational needs. These children generally have a low IQ and will require a lot of educational support.

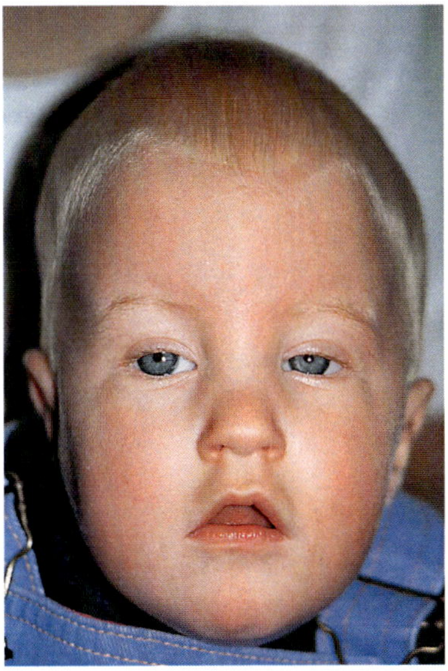

Fig. 8.11 *Typical facies of Prader–Willi syndrome.*
(Reproduced with kind permission from Lissauer T, Clayden G. Illustrated Textbook of Paediatrics, 2nd edn. Edinburgh: Mosby, 2001.)

Can you explain the inheritance pattern of this syndrome?

Prader–Willi and Angelman syndromes are two examples of a type of Mendelian inheritance known as imprinting. Imprinting is when a gene only expresses the copy derived from a parent of a given sex. The Prader–Willi and Angelman syndrome genes are separate but both are located in bands 11–13 of the long arm of chromosome 15 (15q11–13). Normally the paternal copy of the Prader–Willi gene and the maternal copy of the Angelman gene are active. Failure to inherit the particular active gene gives rise to the relevant syndrome. The child may fail to inherit the active gene by one of two methods – either from a de novo deletion, giving rise to a new mutation in the child, or uniparental disomy. Uniparental disomy occurs when a child inherits two copies of a region of a chromosome from one parent and none from the other parent. This can be detected with DNA analysis.

What is the prognosis for this condition?

During adolescence these children frequently develop behavioural problems. In later life, cardiac and respiratory complications arise secondary to obesity and life expectancy is reduced.

ANGELMAN SYNDROME

STEM: Rosie is a 7-year-old girl with profound learning difficulties. Please examine her.

PRESENTATION OF EXAMINATION FINDINGS

Rosie is a 7-year-old girl with an unsteady, jerky, broad-based gait resembling the step of a marionette. She has a happy disposition with frequent

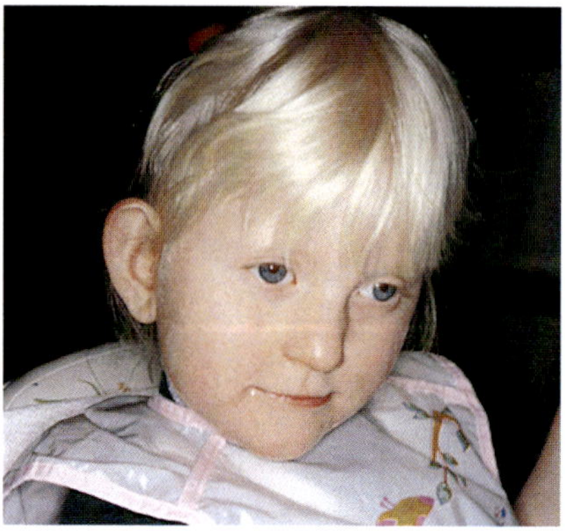

Fig. 8.12 *Angelman syndrome.*
(Reproduced with kind permission from Winrow A P, Gatzoulis M, Supramaniam G. 100 Paediatric Picture Tests. Edinburgh: Churchill Livingstone, 1994.)

outbursts of hand flapping and laughter. She has a typical facial appearance, with fair hair, microcephaly, maxillary hypoplasia with a large mouth and a prominent chin. Rosie has profound impairment of speech.

Thinking pause… ..
Rosie is a little girl with the characteristic features of Angelman syndrome.

Anything else?

I would like to ask the parents if Rosie suffers from epilepsy. Also, I would like to ask about her educational needs as she will require tremendous educational support for her severe learning difficulties.

How is this condition inherited?

Angelman syndrome results from deletion of the maternal copy of a gene on the long arm of chromosome 15 at 15q11–13 in 60% of cases. A small number of cases have paternal disomy for chromosome 15 and at least 20% have normal chromosomes.

KLINEFELTER'S SYNDROME

STEM: Neil is a teenage boy who has always required learning support at school. Over the last 6 months his parents and school teachers have become increasingly concerned about his change in behaviour. His mother has also noticed that he has some breast development and worries that this is causing him great anxiety and feels that this could be the source of his bad behaviour. Please examine him.

PRESENTATION OF EXAMINATION FINDINGS

Neil is a tall and thin 15-year-old adolescent with moderate bilateral gynaecomastia. I would like to plot his height and weight on a growth chart appropriate for his age and sex. I would also like to assess his pubertal development, including testicular volume.

Thinking pause.....
Neil is a boy with Klinefelter's syndrome.

How is this condition inherited?

This is a chromosomal disorder with the karyotype 47XXY and an incidence of 1 in 1000 males. This is due to meiotic non-disjunction with the extra X chromosome coming from the mother in 50% of cases and from the father in 50%. Increasing maternal age is a risk factor. A number of variants exist with more than two X chromosomes and mosaicism commonly occurs.

How does it present?

The children are generally asymptomatic during the preschool years, after which time they may present with behavioural, educational and psychological problems. Intelligence may be normal but is often below average. Puberty may be delayed and some patients may benefit from testosterone replacement. During puberty the oestradiol levels are high and testosterone levels relatively low which may account for the high incidence (80%) of gynaecomastia. These men have small testes and phallus and infertility is common secondary to azoospermia.

What other health problems may these men experience?

Klinefelter's is associated with an increased risk of respiratory disease, varicose veins and haematological and solid malignancies, including leukaemia, breast and mediastinal germ cell tumours.

MARFAN'S SYNDROME

STEM: Nathan is a teenage boy who first presented to the paediatric team at the age of 11 years when he developed a spontaneous pneumothorax. Please examine him.

PRESENTATION OF EXAMINATION FINDINGS

Nathan is a 13-year-old boy with tall stature and an arm span that exceeds his height. He has a long narrow face and a high arched palate. He has

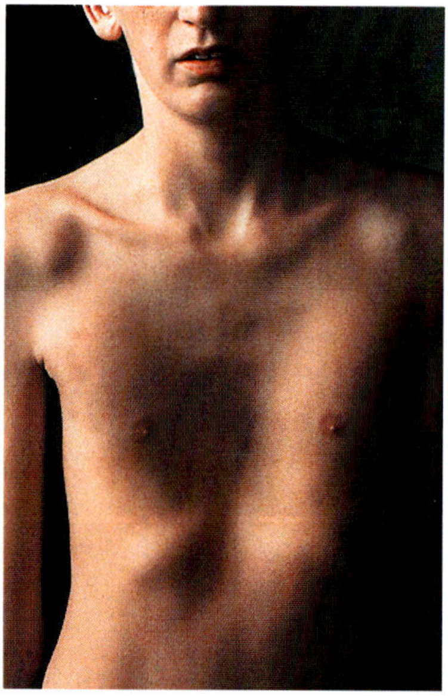

Fig. 8.13 *Marked pectus excavatum.*
(Reproduced with permission from Lissauer T, Roberts G, Foster C, Coren M. Illustrated Self Assessment in Paediatrics. Edinburgh: Mosby, 2001.)

heterochromia of the iris with blue sclerae. He wears glasses to correct for myopia and he has subluxation of the lens upwards and outwards. He has arachnodactyly and hyperextensible joints. Ligamentous laxity demonstrated by opposition of the thumb onto the flexor surface of the forearm, hyperextension of the elbow, knee and fingers. He can also place the palm of his hands on the floor when the knees are extended. Nathan also has a funnel-shaped chest. I would like to plot his height and weight on a growth chart appropriate for his age and sex and to perform a cardiovascular examination.

Thinking pause.....
Nathan is a teenage boy with the characteristic features of Marfan's syndrome.

Why could this not as easily be homocystinuria?

Marfan's syndrome and homocystinuria have a lot of similar features but in homocystinuria the lens is characteristically subluxed downwards and inwards, although the two could be differentiated by examining urine and plasma amino acids for the presence of homocysteine.

A summary of the common features of Marfan's syndrome are shown in Table 8.2. For comparison, the features of homocystinuria are also included.

Table 8.2 Comparison of common features of Marfan's syndrome and homocystinuria

Feature	Marfan's syndrome	Homocystinuria
Incidence	1 in 16 000–60 000	1 in 300 000
Inheritance	Autosomal dominant – chromosome 15	Autosomal recessive
At birth	Usually abnormal	Normal (prenatal Dx possible)
Height	Tall stature: lower >upper segment; arm span >height	Tall stature: lower >upper segment; arm span >height
Hands	Arachnodactyly	Arachnodactyly
Connective tissue	Hernia, scoliosis	Hernia, scoliosis
Joints	Hyperextendable joints	Hyperextendable joints
Eyes	Lens subluxation – upwards and outwards; myopia, retinal detachment, glaucoma, cataract	Lens subluxation – downwards and inwards
Cardiovascular	Mitral valve prolapse and incompetence; aortic valve incompetence and aortic root dilatation	Increased risk of vascular thrombosis
Respiratory	Pneumothorax	
Haematological	Platelet dysfunction	
Intellect	Usually normal	Progressive intellectual decline (70%)

What cardiac features would you expect to find?

Cardiovascular problems are a significant cause of morbidity and mortality in these patients. Degeneration of the media of vessel walls results in dilated valves with aortic incompetence, mitral valve prolapse and regurgitation. Rupture or dissection of an aortic aneurysm may also occur. Consequently, echocardiography monitoring is required.

EHLERS–DANLOS SYNDROME

STEM: Alexander is a teenage boy who has always been 'double-jointed' and has a tendency to bruise easily. Please examine him.

PRESENTATION OF EXAMINATION FINDINGS

Alexander is a teenager with elastic 'raspberry' scars, particularly of the knees and elbows, and he demonstrates hyperextensibility of his joints. He has increased ligamentous laxity in at least five areas including thumb, fingers, elbow, knees and shoulders. Alexander also has multiple bruises over his shins.

Thinking pause.....

Alexander has the characteristic features of a connective tissue disorder. The lack of signs to support a diagnosis of Marfan's syndrome would favour a diagnosis of Ehlers–Danlos syndrome.

What is Ehlers–Danlos syndrome?

Ehlers–Danlos syndrome is the most common inherited connective tissue disorder, characterised by hypermobile joints and atrophic scars. It is also associated with platelet dysfunction and there is a lifelong tendency to excessive bruising and haematoma formation together with increased bleeding and poor wound healing postsurgery. There is no specific treatment.

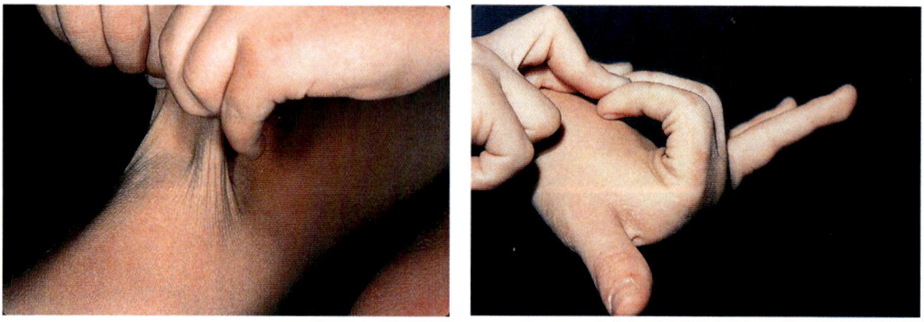

a b

Fig. 8.14 (**a**) *Hyperextensibility of the skin;* (**b**) *joint hypermobility.*
(Reproduced with kind permission from Schachner L A, Hansen R C. Pediatric Dermatology, 3rd edn. Edinburgh: Mosby, 2003.)

There are currently eight different types of EDS recognised with features particular to a specific type. EDS Type IV is characterised by extremely friable arteries that are prone to aneurysm and rupture and are difficult to repair. Consequently it is this group of patients who have an increased risk of cerebrovascular complications. Mutations in the Type V collagen genes account for 50% of the cases of classic EDS, but many other cases are unexplained. It has been suggested that deficiency of the tenascins, which are extracellular matrix proteins highly expressed in connective tissue, may be responsible for a distinct, recessive form of EDS.

GOLDENHAR'S SYNDROME (Oculo-auriculovertebral dysplasia)

STEM: Charlotte was born this morning by an uncomplicated SVD. At birth she was noted to have a funny ear. The midwives have called you to the postnatal wards to review the baby and reassure the mother who is distraught that her baby might not be able to hear. Please examine this baby.

PRESENTATION OF EXAMINATION FINDINGS

Charlotte is a neonate who has a number of dysmorphic facial features. She has mild frontal bossing, facial asymmetry with hemifacial microsomia, and hypomandibulosis. Charlotte has an epibulbar dermoid, unilateral coloboma and atrophy of the iris. Her left ear is abnormal in shape and position, being sited at the angle of the mandible. There are no obvious auricular appendages and pretragal fistulae. She does not have either a cleft lip or palate. Her hearing will require formal testing. Her nostrils are also poorly developed. Her sutures and fontanelles appear normal at present. She has no evidence of spina bifida.

Thinking pause.....
Charlotte is a little girl with the characteristic facial features of Goldenhar's syndrome.

Anything else?
I would like to plot Charlotte's length, weight and OFC on an appropriate centile chart as this condition is often associated with small for gestational age. Although Charlotte does not have a cleft lip or palate, I would also like to enquire as to whether there have been any feeding problems, which may be associated with an anatomically narrow pharyngeal airway.

Why did you mention spina bifida?
This disorder is associated with a number of vertebral anomalies including synostosis, spina bifida, hemivertebrae and cuneiform vertebrae.

How is this condition inherited?
Various inheritance patterns are described but this condition usually occurs sporadically.

How would you manage this patient?

Early detection and management of associated conductive hearing loss is essential. Involvement of the plastic surgery team from birth and repair of clefts when appropriate. Plastic surgery may also play a role in correcting facial asymmetry where possible. Speech therapy is often required. Orthodontic and dental care to correct malocclusion and other dental abnormalities will be necessary. Feeding support may also be required.

What is the prognosis for this condition?

The outlook varies with aetiology and malformations. For those children with no associated chromosomal anomalies or other severe associated malformations, life span is normal. IQ is usually normal, although 5–15% may have reduced intelligence. Understandably, children may develop psychological problems as a result of their facial abnormalities.

TREACHER COLLINS SYNDROME

STEM: Harry is a 1-year-old boy who had problems during the neonatal period establishing feeding. Please examine him.

PRESENTATION OF EXAMINATION FINDINGS

Harry is a 1-year-old boy with maxillary hypoplasia and micrognathia. He has malformed ears with abnormal pinnae. Harry has downward-sloping palpebral fissures with coloboma of the lower eyelids and deficient eyelashes. He does not have evidence of a repaired cleft lip or palate.

Thinking pause.....

Harry is a little boy with the facial features of Treacher Collins syndrome.

Anything else?

I would like to ask if he had any problems sleeping, as in addition to failure to thrive these children can present with sleep apnoea due to maxillary hypoplasia and micrognathia. I would also like to ask about any hearing difficulties he may have, as ear abnormalities are commonly associated with conductive deafness.

How is this condition inherited?

Treacher Collins syndrome is an autosomal dominant condition.

CHARGE ANOMALY

STEM: Robert is 5-year-old boy who has spent a considerable period of his young life in hospital. Please examine him.

PRESENTATION OF EXAMINATION FINDINGS

Robert is a 5-year-old boy who is of short stature. He has bilateral abnormalities of his ears, which appear cup-shaped and anteverted. Robert has bilateral hearing aids. He has a coloboma of the upper eyelid of his left eye. Robert had a midline sternotomy scar in keeping with previous open heart surgery. I would like to plot his height and weight on a growth chart appropriate for his age and sex.

Thinking pause.....
Robert is a young boy with several features of CHARGE syndrome.

Anything else?
I would like to ask his parents whether there were any problems in the early neonatal period. Another feature of this anomaly is choanal atresia, which if bilateral is a neonatal emergency, as babies are obligate nasal breathers.

How would such an emergency have been managed?
Choanal atresia may be confirmed by attempting to pass a fine feeding tube or suction catheter, although use of a radio-opaque dye and radiograph are sometimes necessary. Where the atresia is bilateral the baby requires an oral airway or oral endotracheal intubation followed by surgery. A transnasal or transpalatal approach may be used to open the posterior choanae and patency is maintained by inserting silastic tubes for up to 2 months. Surgical correction of unilateral choanal atresia may be postponed until the child is a few years of age.

FETAL ALCOHOL SYNDROME

STEM: Mohammed is a 3-year-old boy who was referred to the paediatric clinic for further assessment after he failed his 36 months routine child surveillance assessment. Please examine him.

PRESENTATION OF EXAMINATION FINDINGS

Mohammed is a 3-year-old boy with facial dysmorphism. He has a saddle-shaped nose, maxillary hypoplasia, an absent philtrum and a short, thin upper lip. He is small with a disproportionately small head, although I would like to plot his height, weight and head circumference on a growth chart appropriate for his age and sex to confirm this. He is pink in air and has no finger clubbing or evidence of previous cardiac surgery. Mohammed also shows developmental delay in his speech and play and this could be formally tested by performing a developmental assessment.

Thinking pause.....

This is a little boy with the characteristic facies of fetal alcohol syndrome as a result of excessive alcohol ingestion during pregnancy.

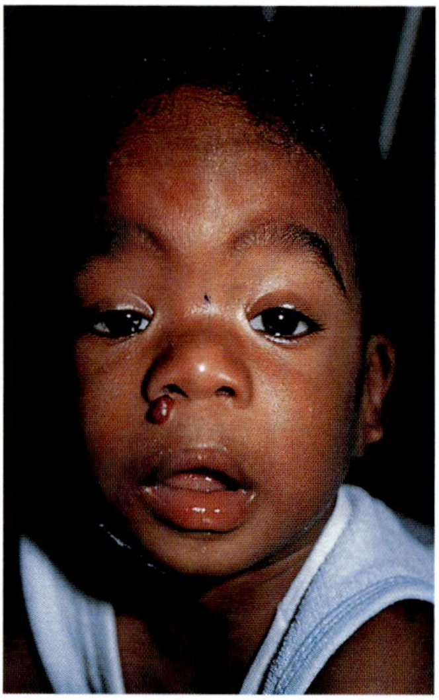

Fig. 8.15 *Characteristic facies of fetal alcohol syndrome with a saddle-shaped nose, maxillary hypoplasia, absent philtrum between the nose and upper lip and a short thin upper lip. This child also has a strawberry naevus below the right nostril.*
(Reproduced with kind permission from Lissauer T, Clayden G. Illustrated Textbook of Paediatrics, 2nd edn. Edinburgh: Mosby, 2001.)

What is fetal alcohol syndrome?

Fetal alcohol syndrome (FAS) is a lifelong yet completely preventable set of physical, mental and neurobehavioral birth defects associated with alcohol consumption during pregnancy. FAS is the leading known cause of learning difficulties and birth defects. Some babies with alcohol-related birth defects, including smaller body size, lower birth weight, and other impairments, do not have all of the classic FAS symptoms. These symptoms are sometimes referred to as fetal alcohol effects (FAE).

Features of FAS include:

- *Growth deficiencies*: small body size and weight, slower than normal development and failure to catch up.
- *Skeletal deformities*: deformed ribs and sternum; curved spine; hip dislocations; bent, fused, webbed, or missing fingers or toes; limited movement of joints; small head.

- *Facial abnormalities*: small eye openings; skin webbing between eyes and base of nose; drooping eyelids; nearsightedness; failure of eyes to move in same direction; short upturned nose; sunken nasal bridge; flat or absent groove between nose and upper lip; thin upper lip; opening in roof of mouth; small jaw; low-set or poorly formed ears.
- *Organ deformities*: heart defects; heart murmurs; genital malformations; kidney and urinary defects.
- *Central nervous system handicaps*: small brain; faulty arrangement of brain cells and connective tissue; learning disabilities – usually mild to moderate but occasionally severe; short attention span; irritability in infancy; hyperactivity in childhood; poor body, hand, and finger coordination.

LAURENCE–MOON–BIEDL SYNDROME

STEM: Kieran is an 8-year-old boy who was failing to cope in mainstream school and was referred to the educational psychologist for further assessment. He was noted to have extra digits and the educational psychologist wondered if there might be some underlying condition to explain his educational difficulties. Please examine him.

PRESENTATION OF EXAMINATION FINDINGS

Kieran is an 8-year-old boy who is tall for his age and very overweight. He does not however have any visible striae. He has bilateral postaxial polydactyly. He has cryptorchidism and micropenis. Kieran has global developmental delay. I would like to plot his height and weight on a growth chart appropriate for his age and sex.

Thinking pause.....
This is a boy with the characteristic appearance of Laurence–Moon–Biedl syndrome.

Anything else?
I would like to look in his eyes for evidence of retinitis pigmentosa.

What is the pathogenesis of this condition?
Laurence–Moon–Biedl syndrome results from a failure of normal embryologic development. The progressive nature suggests a metabolic error that interferes with development and continues after birth in some differentiated cells. It is presumably of autosomal recessive inheritance. There has been no gene identified but genetic counselling is indicated.

What is the prognosis for this condition?
This is a deteriorating handicapping condition due to mental retardation, progressive vision loss and progressive spastic diplegia.

9
THE ENDOCRINE SYSTEM

ENDOCRINE SYSTEM EXAMINATION SUMMARY

GROWTH

Charts: Tanner and Whitehouse; Child Growth Foundation

PUBERTAL STATUS

You will not be expected to do this in the exam but you need to know how to do so

STATURE

You will not be expected to assess this in the exam situation but again you need to know the relevant questions to ask and important examination findings:

- Ask the child to stand
- Inspect for overall height and proportions
- Look for any dysmorphic features
- Offer to measure the height (standing and sitting), weight and head circumference and plot them on a growth chart
- Observe the child's pubertal status as far as possible
- Assess the child's nutritional status
- If parents are with the child make a general observation of their height and appearance
- If the child is short offer to determine the mid-parental height, as illustrated below:

Adult height potential (Child Growth Foundation 1996)

Female: Calculate the adult height potential of a girl as follows:

$$\text{Mid-parental height (MPH, cm)} = \frac{(\text{father's height} + \text{mother's height}) - 7}{2}$$

Male: The adult height potential of a boy is calculated as follows:

$$\text{Mid-parental height (MPH, cm)} = \frac{(\text{father's height} + \text{mother's height}) + 7}{2}$$

Mid-parental centile: Plot the child's adult height potential on the chart and the nearest centile line is the 50th centile, known as the mid-parental centile (MPC).

Target centile range: The child's curve would be expected to follow a centile somewhere between the 9th and 91st centiles (mid-parental height ± 8.5 cm), known as the target centile range (TCR).

ENDOCRINOLOGY SHORT CASES

STEROID TOXICITY

STEM: Jason is a 6-year-old boy who has been admitted on three occasions with seizures during febrile illnesses and on two of those occasions has been found to have hypoglycaemia. He has a past history of asthma.

PRESENTATION OF EXAMINATION FINDINGS

On examination, he has no clinical features of chronic asthma (no hyperinflation, no Harrison's sulcus), there is no wheeze on auscultation and his peak flow rate is 250 l/minute at a time when his height is measured at 103 cm.

Thinking pause .....

This is a boy with a history of asthma but no corroborative physical signs.

Anything else?

He also has short stature. I would like to know his parents' heights in order that I can plot the mid-parental height and the target centile range. I would also like serial measurements of Jason's height to calculate his height velocity. He looks proportionate but I would also like to measure his head circumference and weight and plot these on a centile chart. He is not obviously thin or obese, there are no obvious dysmorphic features and his limbs do not seem short in relation to his body.

He is currently receiving 1000 micrograms per day of inhaled steroids. Could this be relevant?

Yes. High doses of inhaled steroids or topical steroids for eczema can cause adrenal suppression. This could impair his ability to mount a stress response, explaining the hypoglycaemia and seizures during a febrile illness. Febrile convulsions are unusual beyond the age of 5 years. Corticosteroid therapy may also be contributing to his short stature.

What further investigations would you like to undertake?

Blood for urea and electrolytes may show a low plasma sodium, a raised plasma potassium and a slightly raised plasma urea in children with adrenal suppression. However, a dynamic adrenal test is required for definitive diagnosis. This requires baseline measurements of cortisol and then the administration of ACTH. The child's cortisol response to this exogenous ACTH challenge is then measured.

Post script

Jason underwent a short Synacthen test which showed a low baseline cortisol at 9.00 a.m. of 80 nmol/l. A single dose of tetracosactrin intravenously of 250 micrograms was then given and repeat plasma cortisol samples were obtained at 30 and 60 minutes after tetracosactrin injection. The 30 minute sample showed an increase to 150 nmol/l and the 60 minute sample a further increase to 170 nmol/l. This is a subnormal response. The normal increment is ≥200 nmol/l, the normal peak is ≥500 nmol/l and the baseline 9.00 a.m. cortisol is usually above 200 nmol/l. Lung function tests showed Jason to have normal forced vital capacity and forced expiratory volume in 1 second. His inhaled steroids were gradually withdrawn, his mother was given a steroid card to carry and Jason was prescribed 10 mg hydrocortisone tablets to take three times a day if he became unwell.

Following cessation of his inhaled steroids, his height gradually increased from the 0.4th centile to the 9th centile.

PSEUDOHYPOPARATHYROIDISM

STEM: Donald is a 13-year-old boy who had been previously well but presented with diplopia and muscle spasms in his hands and thighs. His parents are consanguineous. On examination he had obvious carpopedal spasm but Chvostek's sign was negative. Please can you examine his hands.

PRESENTATION OF EXAMINATION FINDINGS

Donald has short fourth and fifth metacarpals.

What is the most likely cause for the acute condition Donald presented with?

The presentation is most in keeping with hypocalcaemic tetany.

In an adolescent girl, the commonest cause for this would be hyperventilation as part of a panic attack. The patient may also report symptoms of palpitations, headache, nausea, sweating and indeed may faint.

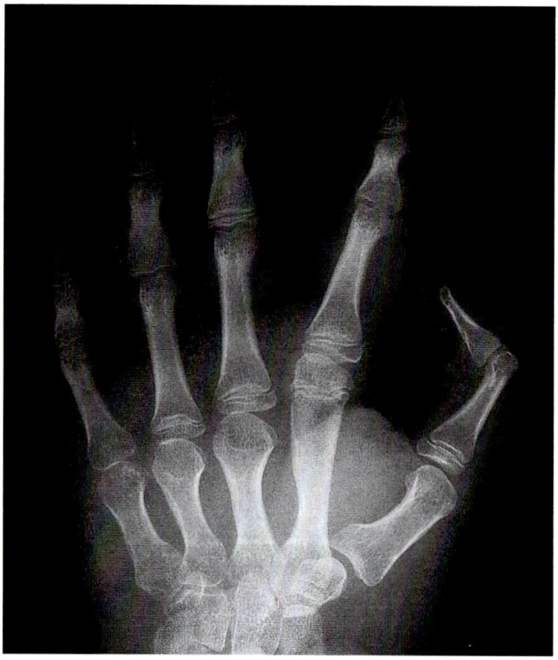

Fig. 9.1 *Pseudohypoparathyroidism with short third to fifth metacarpals and cone epiphyses.*
(Reproduced with kind permission from Wales J K H, Wit J-M, Rogol A D. Pediatric Endocrinology and Growth, 2nd edn. Edinburgh: Saunders, 2003.)

Hyperventilation leads to hypocapnia and the respiratory alkalosis reduces the circulating free calcium concentration. Hypocalcaemic tetany due to hyperventilation can be reversed by encouraging the child or teenager to re-breathe into a paper bag so that carbon dioxide levels rise and return within the normal range. In an adolescent boy, panic attacks are less common and indeed on examination there was no evidence of tachypnoea or hyperventilation.

What initial investigations would you undertake?

Bloods should be taken for calcium, albumin, phosphate, alkaline phosphatase and magnesium. These showed that Donald's blood calcium level was 1.09 mmol/l (normal range 2.1–2.6), with an albumin of 41 g/l (normal), and a phosphate elevated at 1.97 mmol/l (normal range 1.0–1.8). Alkaline phosphatase was 395 units/l (normal range 100–400). His 25-hydroxycholecalciferol was low at 7 nmol/l (normal range 10–75) and his magnesium was also low at 0.69 mmol/l (normal range 0.7–1.0).

How would you treat Donald acutely?

Donald was given 10% calcium gluconate 10 ml over 5 minutes with ECG monitoring. Six hours later and after two such boluses, carpopedal spasm was still present. A further bolus was therefore given, after which his cramps disappeared and he was able to extend his fingers.

On subsequent examination we also noted, as you correctly pointed out, that he has short metacarpals. Blood was therefore taken for a parathyroid hormone level which was elevated at 251 ng/l (reference range 12–72).

What is the most likely diagnosis now?

These investigations showing decreased calcium, elevated phosphate and elevated parathyroid hormone are consistent with pseudohypoparathyroidism. Despite the elevated secretion of parathyroid hormone by the parathyroid gland, there is end-organ insensitivity and hypocalcaemia results. Further outpatient treatment was with alfacalcidol 35 ng/kg/day and calcium supplements 400 mg tablets, four tablets per day. An autoantibody screen was negative, skull X-ray showed no intracranial calcification and hand X-ray showed no obvious osteodystrophy.

With this treatment there were no further episodes of tetany over the succeeding year of follow-up and no muscle cramps but lethargy, particularly with exercise, remained a problem and Donald described numb finger tips in cold weather.

Background

End-organ resistance due to receptor or post-receptor abnormalities is more common than true hypoparathyroidism. PTH resistance can arise due to hypomagnesaemia and rickets (due to low 1,25-dihydroxyvitamin D levels). However, receptor or post-receptor defects of response to PTH are commoner and were first described by Albright and therefore sometimes termed Albright's hereditary osteodystrophy. Parathyroid hormone acts on the renal tubule to cause phosphaturia and, therefore, resistance to parathyroid hormone leads to phosphate retention and, in parallel with this, hypocalcaemia.

- *Type 1 pseudohypoparathyroidism*: There is symptomatic hypocalcaemia in mid-childhood on a background of mental retardation and characteristic phenotypic features (as originally described by Albright) including short stature, obesity, round face, short neck and marked metacarpal and metatarsal shortening (especially the fourth and fifth metacarpals). Following administration of PTH, there is no phosphaturic response and a blunted urinary cyclic AMP increase compared to normal.
- *Type 2 pseudohypoparathyroidism*: In this rarer form, there is no phosphaturic response to PTH but urinary cyclic AMP response is normal. This suggests the defect is due to an intracellular abnormality beyond cyclic AMP generation. The clinical manifestations are very variable. Children who have the phenotypic appearance but do not have the biochemical abnormalities are referred to as having pseudopseudohypoparathyroidism.

PTH activates the adenylate cyclase system via the G protein and G proteins mediate numerous transmembrane hormone responses including LH, GH and TSH. Therefore, abnormalities of other hormones have been described in these patients. Donald was screened with thyroid function tests which showed a normal TSH of 2.5 mIU/l (normal range 0.4–6.3) but a free T4 of 11.2 pmol/l (at the lower limit of the normal range of 11–26). These results are not in keeping with an abnormality of TSH release and no thyroxine treatment was started.

SHORT STATURE

STEM: John is a 16-year-old boy who is being teased at school because he is short. Please would you examine him.

PRESENTATION OF EXAMINATION FINDINGS

John is a 16-year-old boy with a weight of 52 kg and a height of 152 cm, both of which lie just below the 3rd centile on the growth chart. He does not have any dysmorphic features. He does not have any clinical signs of an underactive thyroid and does not have a goitre. He does not have any axillary hair and shows only early signs of pubic hair development. I have not examined his genitalia.

Thinking pause.....

John is a very well 16-year-old boy with short stature and lack of virilisation, although I have not formally assessed pubertal staging. The most likely cause of this is constitutional delay of growth and puberty. I would like to ask him if he has a history of headaches and visual disturbance and I would assess his visual fields and fundii to ensure he does not have a craniopharyngioma. It would also be important to determine whether he had any symptoms suggestive of a chronic illness, for example bowel disturbance, productive cough.

What important investigations might be helpful here?

A lateral skull X-ray would be helpful to look for suprasellar calcification present in 90% of craniopharyngiomas, but a CT scan should be considered. Thyroid function is mandatory in any patient who presents with short stature. In general patients who are short and thin with decreased subcutaneous fat may have a chronic illness whereas patients who are short with increased subcutaneous fat may have an endocrine disorder, for example hypothyroidism or growth hormone deficiency.

How would you confirm the diagnosis?

Diagnosis of CDGP is a clinical diagnosis. Bone age estimation may be helpful, this would be significantly delayed. Management is dependent upon whether the patient is in early established puberty or entirely prepubertal. This is best determined by assessment of testicular volume with early established puberty being present if the testicles are 4 ml or greater in volume.

How would you manage a 16 year old with CDGP who is in early established puberty?

In general there are three options here:

1. No intervention, accepting that this is a timing problem and that as puberty progresses, a growth spurt will happen and he will achieve his expected final height as assessed from parental heights, albeit at an age much later than his peers.
2. If short stature is the main problem then a trial of growth hormone therapy should be considered.
3. If lack of virilisation is the major concern then a course of oxandrolone for 3–6 months should be considered. Some endocrinologists use both growth hormone and oxandrolone with careful monitoring.

GOITRE

STEM: You are given a growth chart which demonstrates a decreasing height velocity over the past 12 months.

PRESENTATION OF EXAMINATION FINDINGS

Jessica is a 12-year-old girl with a diffuse, solid, non-fluctuant swelling on the anterior aspect of her neck in the midline. The swelling elevates when

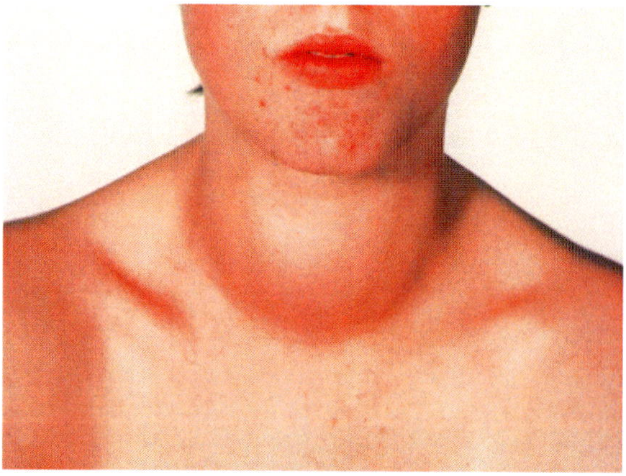

Fig. 9.2 *Goitre.*

she swallows some water but does not elevate when she protrudes her tongue. She is relatively short and overweight, although I would like to plot her height and weight on a growth chart appropriate for her age and sex. She has no evidence of pubertal development.

Thinking pause.....
Jessica is a 12-year-old girl with short stature and a goitre. I think she has hypothyroidism.

Anything else?
I would like to assess her reflexes for delayed relaxation.

What questions would you like to ask in the history?
I would like to ask whether she has any problems with feeling cold and more tired than usual. I would ask Jessica about her appetite and whether she has noticed herself gain weight over the last few months. Also I would like to ask her whether she has any problems with constipation, and whether she has noticed any change in her skin or hair texture recently. I would like to ask her parents whether Jessica's teacher has made any comment about any deterioration in concentration at school. I would also like to ask whether Jessica has any recent history of hip discomfort or has been limping, as it is not uncommon for these children to present with a slipped upper femoral epiphysis, associated with secondary epiphyseal dysgenesis.

What is likely to be the underlying thyroid disorder?
The most common cause of this is autoimmune thyroiditis, which is more prevalent in girls. Treatment of this condition is with thyroxine. This condition is often associated with other autoimmune conditions, such as diabetes mellitus, particularly in children with Down's syndrome or Turner's syndrome.

HYPERTHYROIDISM

STEM: This 14-year-old girl presents with her parents because they have noticed that she has a swelling in her neck. Please examine.

PRESENTATION OF EXAMINATION FINDINGS

Judith is a 14-year-old girl with a palpable goitre and on auscultation a bruit can be heard. She has exophthalmos with lid retraction and lid lag but no evidence of external ophthalmoplegia. Judith has warm and sweaty hands with a fine tremor at rest. She has a mild tachycardia but no heart murmur present. Judith also has several areas of vitiligo. Judith is a tall slim girl and I would like to plot her height and weight on a growth chart appropriate for her age and sex.

Thinking pause.....
Judith is a teenage girl with a palpable goitre and clinical features in keeping with a diagnosis of thyrotoxicosis.

Anything else?
I would like to measure her blood pressure, as this condition may be associated with hypertension. I would also like to assess her muscle strength to look for proximal muscle weakness.

What is likely to be the underlying thyroid disorder?
The most likely diagnosis is Graves' disease, which is the most common cause of thyrotoxicosis and is three times more common in females, presenting particularly during the teenage years. The clinical features are similar to those seen in adults (summarised in Box 9.1).

How would you confirm the diagnosis?
Measurement of thyroid hormones would reveal elevated levels of thyroxine and/or tri-iodothyronine together with low TSH levels. Antithyroid antibodies are also usually present.

How would you manage this patient?
The first line of treatment is generally medical, with drugs such as carbimazole or propyl-thiouracil, which block the synthesis of thyroid hormone. If patients are symptomatic β-blockers may also be added in. Medical therapy is administered over a 2-year period to achieve control of thyrotoxicosis, although resolution of signs, particularly exophthalmos and lid lag, may not resolve completely. Once medical therapy is discontinued up to 75% of patients will relapse and management of these patients may involve reinstitution of medical therapy, radio-iodine or surgery. Radio-iodine is a simple method of treatment and has not been shown to be associated with genetic damage or malignancy. Permanent remission is seen

Box 9.1 Features of Graves' disease

History

- Anxiety, restlessness
- Thin, weight loss (despite increased appetite)
- Heat intolerance, sweating
- Learning difficulties/behavioural problems
- Rapid growth in height (advanced in bone-age)

Examination

- General: hyperpigmentation, vitiligo and very rarely pretibial myxoedema
- Hands: fine tremor, warm and sweaty, tachycardia
- Neck: goitre (bruit)
- Eye signs (not always present):
  - — exophthalmos
  - — lid retraction: the eyelid fails to bisect a cord across the iris therefore the sclerae are visible above the iris
  - — lid lag: ask the child to follow the movements of your finger slowly upwards and downwards – the sclera becomes visible above the iris on downward gaze as the eyelid is slow to follow the movement of the eye
  - — rarely external ophthalmoplegia involving lateral or superior rectus muscles
- Cardiovascular:
  - — hyperactive praecordium and there may be an ejection systolic murmur
  - — blood pressure is elevated, with an increased pulse pressure
- Neurological: proximal muscle weakness

after subtotal thyroidectomy. These patients often subsequently develop hypothyroidism and require thyroxine replacement, therefore follow-up is necessary.

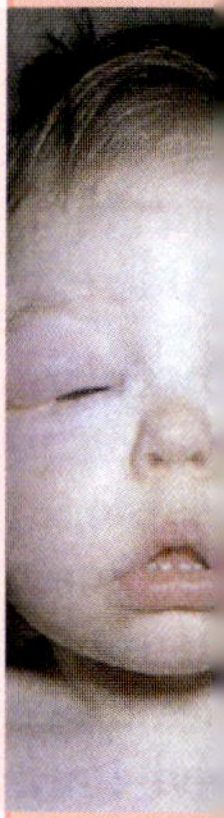

10 THE RENAL SYSTEM

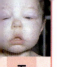

RENAL SYSTEM EXAMINATION SUMMARY

Examination of the kidneys is obviously part of the abdominal system (see Ch. 9) but once renal pathology is suspected it is important to be vigilant for other clues, which may point towards the underlying diagnosis.

- *Height* and *weight* are always essential – short stature, anorexia
- *Skeletal assessment* – renal osteodystrophy (renal rickets)
- *Abdominal scars* – Rutherford Morrison scar for renal transplant (don't forget renal biopsy scars)
- *Peritoneal dialysis* – catheter in situ
- *AV fistulae* – haemodialysis
- *Dentition* – immunosuppression
- *Anaemia* – reduced erythropoietin and metabolites causing marrow toxicity
- *Urinalysis* – blood, protein, glucose
- *Hypertension*
- *Eyes* – cataracts (inborn error of metabolism)

RENAL SHORT CASES

PALPABLE RENAL MASS

STEM: Kathi is a girl of 4 years and 10 months who has a 3-month history of pain below the umbilicus associated with burning dysuria and nocturnal enuresis on two occasions. She has also had daytime urge incontinence but no haematuria. She had previously been dry by day from the age of 2 years and dry by night from the age of 3 years. The results of a urine sample led the GP to prescribe a course of trimethoprim antibiotics. There is no family history of renal problems. Please examine her abdomen.

PRESENTATION OF EXAMINATION FINDINGS

Kathi is a 4-year-old girl who is bright and alert and comfortable at rest. She is pink and well nourished. Her abdomen is soft and non-tender. She has no hepatomegaly or splenomegaly but I can palpate the lower pole of her left kidney, although her right kidney is not palpable. She has normal bowel sounds. I would like to measure her blood pressure.

Thinking pause .....

This is a girl with a history of urinary tract infection and a palpable renal mass. I believe this to be a kidney rather than spleen because I cannot get above the mass, I cannot palpate a notch and the mass is ballotable on bimanual examination.

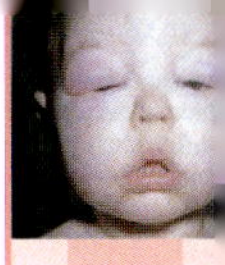

What are the causes of a renal mass?

There are a number of causes of a renal mass, including malignancy, hydronephrosis and polycystic kidneys (Box 10.1).

In hydronephrosis, features that help to determine the level of obstruction include:

- No megaureter – PUJ obstruction
- Megaureter – VUJ obstruction or VUR
- Large bladder – bladder outlet obstruction
- Prune belly syndrome.

A mass arising outside the urinary tract may also cause obstruction of the urinary tract.

What further investigations would you recommend?

A repeat urine sample should be obtained to ensure that the infection has been cleared. Urinalysis should be undertaken in clinic and the urine sent for microscopy, culture and sensitivity. In terms of urinary tract infection in a girl of almost 5 years, further investigation would include a renal ultrasound scan to check that two kidneys are present, that the kidneys are smooth in outline without scarring and that there is no dilatation of the upper renal tract. Renal ultrasound scanning can miss abnormalities of the

Box 10.1 Causes of a palpable renal mass

Intrarenal

- Solid:
  - — Wilms' tumour
  - — renal vein thrombosis (usually haematuria)
  - — benign nephroma (rare neonatal problem)
  - — horseshoe kidney
  - — grafted kidney in the iliac fossa
- Cystic:
  - — hydronephrosis (due to reflux or anatomical obstruction)
  - — single cyst (benign renal cyst)
  - — multicystic:*
    - a. dysplastic kidney
    - b. polycystic disease – infantile (autosomal recessive) onset; adult (autosomal dominant) onset

Extrarenal

- An adrenal mass (e.g. neuroblastoma) is difficult to distinguish clinically
- A left 'renal' mass may be the spleen

* Nephronophthisis, medullary sponge kidney and congenital nephrotic syndrome are other causes of multicystic kidney on USS but rarely present as abdominal mass.

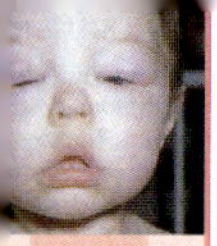

lower renal tract and mild degrees of vesicoureteric reflux. However, this is less significant in a girl of 5 years since most severe reflux presents before this age and evidence suggests that most of the damage to the kidneys occurs in the first few years of life. A micturating cystogram would, therefore, not be justified. A DMSA isotope scan could also be undertaken to look for evidence of scarring.

If the ultrasound scan showed that the left kidney was significantly enlarged and that this was due to hydronephrosis, then further investigation using intravenous isotopic indirect cystography would be indicated. This allows detection of vesicoureteric reflux in an older child who is able to micturate voluntarily.

If renal ultrasound scan showed that the left kidney was significantly enlarged and that this was due to a solid renal mass, the most likely diagnosis is Wilms' tumour or neuroblastoma. In the assessment of a solid renal mass, in addition to abdominal USS, the following investigations would be appropriate:

- Height and weight
- FBC
- U&E, creatinine, calcium, phosphate
- LFT
- Clotting studies
- Screen for increased urinary catecholamines (found in 90% of neuroblastoma cases); 'spot' sample for VMA:creatinine ratio – diagnostic if elevated but false negatives occur – 24 hour collection for VMA is more sensitive
- CXR.

Further investigation may include bone scan, IVP, CT (if Wilms' tumour is suspected) and bone marrow biopsy (if neuroblastoma is diagnosed). Definitive histological diagnosis requires biopsy of mass.

Post script

On ultrasound scanning the right kidney measured 7.1 cm and the left kidney 7.9 cm. The measurement of the left kidney was between 1 and 2 standard deviations for Kathi's height and both kidneys were smooth in outline with no evidence of scarring and no dilatation of the pelvicalyceal systems and ureters.

Each kidney normally moves slightly with respiration. The right kidney normally lies at a slightly lower level than the left kidney, and the lower pole of the right kidney may be palpated in the right lumbar region at the end of deep inspiration in a thin child or a wasted child with poorly developed abdominal musculature. The kidney develops embryologically as a pelvic organ and only later ascends in the abdomen to take up its final position. Rarely is the ascent arrested. A horseshoe kidney and other congenital abnormalities of the kidney may also be palpable. A horseshoe kidney is associated with Turner's syndrome.

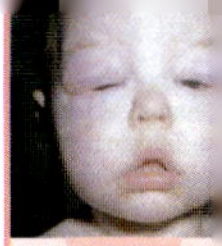

NEPHROTIC SYNDROME

STEM: Alan is a 2-year-old boy who presents with a 2-week history of increasing facial swelling. He has been treated by his GP with oral antihistamines for a presumed allergic reaction. Please examine him.

PRESENTATION OF EXAMINATION FINDINGS

Alan is a 2-year-old boy with obvious periorbital oedema, and in addition he has generalised oedema and in particular pitting oedema of his legs up to the knees. He appears to have abdominal distension but his abdomen is soft and non-tender and he has no organomegaly. He also has bilateral scrotal swelling. It is difficult to ascertain clinically whether he has ascites. I would like to measure his blood pressure.

Thinking pause.....

Alan is a 2-year-old boy with generalised oedema who is otherwise well.

What is the differential diagnosis?

Starling's law regulates the equilibration of fluid across capillaries between the intravascular space and the extravascular space. The extravascular space is made up of intracellular fluid and interstitial fluid and it is an increase in interstitial fluid which gives rise to clinical oedema. In theory, therefore, oedema can arise due to an increase in intravascular pressure or a reduction in intravascular oncotic pressure. It is the proteins within the circulating plasma which contribute most to the intravascular oncotic pressure and it is this oncotic pressure which opposes the hydrostatic pressure tending to force fluid out of the capillaries.

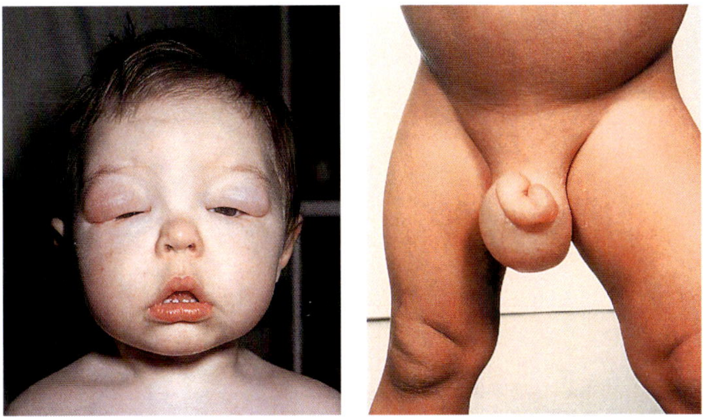

a b

Fig. 10.1 (**a**) *Facial oedema in nephrotic syndrome;* (**b**) *gross oedema of the scrotum and legs as well as abdominal distension from ascites.*
(Reproduced with kind permission from Lissauer T, Clayden G. Illustrated Textbook of Paediatrics, 2nd edn. Edinburgh: Mosby, 2001.)

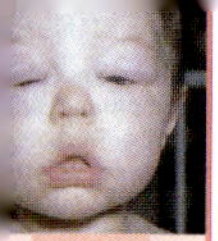

In adults, an example of generalised oedema arising due to increased intravascular pressure is the ankle, sacral and scrotal oedema seen in right ventricular failure. However, in children, generalised oedema is very rarely due to cardiac failure. In children, localised oedema may arise due to increased intravascular pressure (e.g. a malignant mass in the abdomen obstructing venous return from the leg) but generalised oedema is almost always due to hypoproteinaemia. Hypoproteinaemia can arise due to one of four causes:

1. Worldwide the commonest cause is kwashiorkor due to a protein-deficient diet. Growth is stunted and there is a pot belly due to ascites.
2. Liver failure: in end-stage liver failure, the liver is no longer able to synthesise albumin.
3. Protein-losing enteropathy: see Box 10.2 for causes of protein-losing enteropathy.
4. Hypoalbuminaemia arising as a result of severe proteinuria: causes of proteinuria are listed in Box 10.3. Proteinuria arising from tubular damage is occasionally sufficient to result in a nephrotic syndrome but most cases of nephrotic syndrome are due to glomerular proteinuria.

Box 10.2 Causes of protein-losing enteropathy

Increased mucosal permeability to protein

- Hypertrophic gastritis
- Eosinophilic gastroenteritis
- Polyposis
- Inflammatory disease:
  - — Crohn's disease
  - — ulcerative colitis
  - — enterocolitis
  - — pseudomembranous colitis
  - — radiation enteritis
  - — graft-versus-host disease
  - — autoimmune enteropathy
- Coeliac disease
- Oesophagitis

Altered lymph flow

- Primary intestinal lymphangiectasia
- Secondary intestinal lymphangiectasia:
  - — congestive cardiac failure
  - — constrictive pericarditis
  - — lymphoma
  - — tuberculous adenitis
  - — volvulus

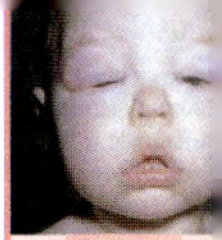

Box 10.3 Causes of proteinuria

Intermittent proteinuria

- Postural (orthostatic)
- Non-postural:
  - — exercise
  - — fever
  - — anatomic abnormalities, e.g. urinary tract
  - — glomerular lesions, e.g. Berger's disease

Persistent proteinuria

- Glomerular:
  - — isolated asymptomatic proteinuria
  - — damage to glomerular basement membrane, e.g. acute or chronic glomerulonephritis
  - — loss or reduction of basement membrane anionic charge, e.g. minimal change and congenital nephrosis
  - — increased permeability in residual nephrons, e.g. chronic renal failure
- Tubular:
  - — hereditary, e.g. cystinosis, Wilson's disease, Lowe's syndrome, proximal tubular acidosis, galactosaemia
  - — acquired, e.g. interstitial nephritis, acute tubular necrosis, post-renal transplantation, pyelonephritis, vitamin D intoxication, penicillamine, heavy metal poisoning (gold, lead, mercury, etc.), analgesic abuse, drugs

What further investigations would you undertake?

The simplest investigation is to look for proteinuria. If heavy proteinuria is present, then the oedema is most likely due to hypoalbuminaemia secondary to urine protein loss. Hence liver disease and protein-losing enteropathy can be discounted.

Dipstick urinalysis of Alan's urine in the out-patient clinic showed ++++ of protein.

What can you tell me about nephrotic syndrome?

Nephrotic syndrome is characterised by a triad of:

1. heavy proteinuria (greater than 40 mg/h/m^2 or a urinary protein to creatinine ratio greater than 200 mg/mmol)
2. hypoalbuminaemia (less than 25 g/l)
3. oedema.

Nephrotic syndrome is a rare disorder (incidence about 2 per 100 000 population) and may be congenital or acquired. Histologically, 80% of non-congenital cases will be due to minimal change disease and 90% of children with minimal change nephrotic syndrome will respond to oral steroids within 7–10 days. However, 75% of those who respond initially will have a

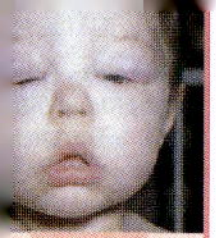

subsequent relapse (recurrence of proteinuria) and about one-third will suffer from frequent relapses.

What further investigations would you undertake?

- FBC
- U&E
- Hepatitis B surface antigen
- Varicella zoster and measles immune status: this is because chickenpox and measles are major threats to the child once they start steroid therapy. Zoster immune globulin should be given if there is chickenpox exposure while taking high-dose prednisolone.

If the clinical features are not typical, or the child is not steroid responsive, then further tests should be undertaken as follows:

- ASO titre
- serum complement
- antinuclear factor.

Nephrotic syndrome can also arise secondary to Henoch–Schönlein purpura, connective tissue disorders such as SLE, drugs and heavy metal poisoning, sickle cell disease and amyloidosis.

What are the possible complications of nephrotic syndrome?

1. Hypovolaemia, often associated with abdominal pain.
2. Nephrotic children are at greater risk of arterial and venous thrombosis. This is probably because of the loss of antithrombin III as part of the proteinuria and the risk is greatest when the child is hypovolaemic and haemoconcentrated. Cerebral and renal vein thromboses are the most serious complications.
3. Infection. Pneumococcal peritonitis is the major risk. Oral penicillin should be prescribed in the oedematous child as prophylaxis. If peritonitis is suspected, abdominal paracentesis should be undertaken and broad-spectrum antibiotics started to cover Gram-negative organisms as well as pneumococci.
4. Hyperlipidaemia.

What are the indications for renal biopsy?

1. Unusual features such as a very young child (under 1 year), relatively old child (more than 12 years) or persistent, heavy haematuria, hypocomplementaemia, hypotension or renal failure.
2. The nephrotic syndrome does not respond to a therapeutic trial of 28 days of prednisolone in which case the underlying histology may be focal segmental (10%), membranoproliferative (8%), mesangioproliferative (2.5%) or membranous (1.5%). Further immunosuppression may be required with drugs such as cyclophosphamide and this should not be embarked on without histological confirmation at renal biopsy.

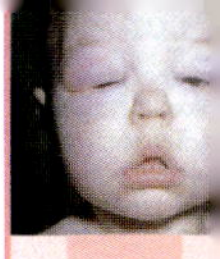

CHRONIC RENAL FAILURE

STEM: Jonathan is a 3-year-old child who first presented over a year ago with Henoch–Schönlein purpura. In addition to the classic palpable purpuric rash, at presentation he had haematuria and proteinuria. He has now been referred back by his GP because he has had two further relapses of Henoch–Schönlein purpura and his parents think that he is more tired with decreased appetite. His height was on the 50th centile at presentation over a year ago and is now on the 25th centile in your clinic. Please examine him.

PRESENTATION OF EXAMINATION FINDINGS

Jonathan is a young boy with pallor but otherwise there are no specific abnormalities.

Thinking pause.....

The most likely cause of anaemia in this age group is iron deficiency anaemia due to a poor diet. I would like to check his full blood count and blood film. (However, although the full blood count shows a haemoglobin of 10 g/dl, there is a normochromic/normocytic picture.)

What other cause for his symptoms should you consider?

Seventy per cent of children with Henoch–Schönlein purpura have haematuria (mainly microscopic) and/or proteinuria early in the course of their illness. In most cases this resolves. However, some present with frank haematuria and some have a persistent nephritis or a nephrotic syndrome. However, of all children presenting with Henoch–Schönlein purpura, only 1–3% will develop chronic renal failure.

Chronic renal failure is relatively rare in childhood. Children may present with non-specific signs such as lethargy, poor appetite, nausea, anaemia, growth failure or urinary symptoms such as polyuria or a secondary enuresis. Chronic renal failure can be congenital or acquired. The commonest causes in the UK are as follows.

1. Progressive glomerulonephritis (25% of chronic renal failure in childhood) as in severe Henoch–Schönlein disease or atypical haemolytic uraemic syndrome.
2. Renal scarring (25%) possibly as a result of recurrent urinary tract infection in the presence of vesicoureteric reflux.
3. Hereditary or familial nephropathy (15%), e.g. polycystic kidney disease, Alport's syndrome (hereditary nephritis with deafness), cystinosis.
4. Congenital hypoplasia/dysplasia (15%). The majority of children with hypoplastic/dysplastic kidneys have presented in the past in older childhood with growth failure, anorexia or an acute crisis precipitated by infection. However, more recently, antenatal diagnosis has led to an

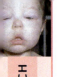

Table 10.1 Stages of chronic renal failure

Stage	GFR (ml/min/1.73 m^2)	Features
Mild	50–75	Asymptomatic
Moderate	25–50	Metabolic abnormalities
Severe	<25	Progressive growth failure
End-stage renal failure	<10	Require renal replacement therapy

increasing number of children with renal tract malformations being detected before symptoms develop.

5. The other 20% of chronic renal failure presentations in childhood are due to multisystem disease (e.g. immunological diseases and kidney tumours).

The stage of chronic renal failure can be defined by measurement of the glomerular filtration rate (GFR) (Table 10.1). However, it should be noted that chronic renal failure is usually asymptomatic and urea and creatinine concentrations in the blood will remain within the normal range until the GFR has fallen to 25% of normal. If often seems confusing that, unlike acute renal failure, chronic renal failure is accompanied by polyuria rather than oliguria because of the continued production of poor quality urine and as a result thirst and nocturia may also ensue.

What further investigations would you undertake?

1. Measure the blood pressure
2. Urinalysis
3. FBC and ferritin or zinc protoporphyrin for iron status
4. U&E, creatinine, bicarbonate, albumin and total protein
5. Calcium, phosphate and alkaline phosphatase as renal osteodystrophy is a complication; there may be secondary hyperparathyroidism
6. Left wrist X-ray for bone age and again for evidence of renal osteodystrophy
7. 24-hour urine collection for creatinine clearance is too unreliable. A more accurate GFR is best performed using a radionuclide method such as chromium 51 EDTA or 99 technetium DTPA. GFR can also be approximately assessed as:

$$\text{GFR (ml/min/1.73 m}^2) = \frac{38 \times \text{height (cm)}}{\text{plasma creatinine in } \mu\text{mol/l}}$$

   However, a 24 hour urine collection should be undertaken for urine volume, sodium and protein excretion.

8. Ultrasound of the urinary tract.

End-stage renal failure is defined as the stage at which dialysis and renal transplantation are required. This is usually at a GFR of less than

10 ml/ min/1.73 m^2. Peritoneal dialysis is preferred to haemodialysis in children but renal transplantation is the best mode of renal replacement therapy for children and adolescents in the long term. At all ages paediatric renal transplant recipients have better survival than dialysis patients of the same age. Transplantation also offers the best option in terms of avoiding physical and psychological stigmatisation in older childhood and adolescence. In the UK, 1-year graft survival rates of 80% for cadaveric renal transplantation and 90% for live donor grafts are quoted. 10-year survival rates for grafts of 50% have been reported.

POST-RENAL TRANSPLANT

STEM: Ruth is an 8-year-old girl who had a renal transplant 3 months ago. She presents acutely with fever and non-specific symptoms of lethargy, myalgia and arthralgia. Her brother has recently had a flu-like illness and her parents thought Ruth had the same illness but she has now developed a persistent cough. Please examine her and present your assessment of the problem.

PRESENTATION OF EXAMINATION FINDINGS

On examination Ruth has a tinge of jaundice affecting her sclerae and tachypnoea of 36 per minute. There are inspiratory crepitations audible throughout both lung fields but no wheeze. The grafted kidney is palpable in the right iliac fossa and is tender. She has haematuria and proteinuria on urinalysis.

Thinking pause.....

Children who have had a renal transplant are prone to a number of complications (see Box 10.4). However, of these infections the most common cause of death during the first year after renal transplantation is cytomegalovirus infection. The risk of CMV infection has been reduced by prophylactic use of antiviral drugs, administration of CMV antibody negative blood products and selection of seronegative organ donors. Other infections which must be considered are urinary tract infection (most common in the first month after transplantation), herpes simplex infection, varicella zoster infection, Epstein–Barr virus infection, *Pneumocystis jiroveci* (formerly *P. carinii*), *Aspergillus*, *Candida* and viral hepatitis. The combination of fever, cough and tachypnoea suggests pneumonitis. If the jaundice is unconjugated it could be a haemolytic process due to drug therapy but if a mixed conjugated and unconjugated pattern exists it probably points to viral hepatitis. The tenderness of the grafted kidney suggests graft rejection is a possibility. (Blood tests confirm a mixed conjugated and unconjugated hyperbilirubinaemia with raised transaminases, and neutropenia.)

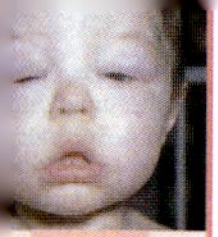

Box 10.4 Post-transplantation complications in paediatric patients

- Acute tubular necrosis
- Rejection reaction
- Technical – vascular, urologic
- Recurrence of original renal disease
- Drug toxicity – immunosuppressives, antibiotics
- Infection – particularly viral, systemic; wound or urinary tract infection
- Bleeding
- Pancreatitis
- Lymphocele
- Urinoma
- Bowel obstruction

How would you manage this child?

Blood should be taken for acute CMV titres and urine collected to look for CMV on culture. However, this will take time and given that there is 5–10% mortality in CMV infection in immunosuppressed patients, treatment must be started empirically. Broad-spectrum antibiotics should be started to cover the possibility of a bacterial pneumonia but in addition antiviral treatment with ganciclovir and anti-CMV immunoglobulin intravenously should be initiated. Direct tissue damage by CMV may result in graft loss but CMV disease may also trigger a rejection reaction. Unfortunately, immunosuppression must usually be discontinued in systemic CMV infection (lung, brain, liver). *Pneumocystis jiroveci* is less likely in Ruth's case since all renal transplant patients receive prophylactic co-trimoxazole (Septrin) which has greatly reduced the incidence of this disease in immunosuppressed patients.

How may Ruth have acquired cytomegalovirus infection?

CMV is a common childhood infection transmitted by direct person-to-person contact. Transmission can occur via saliva, breast milk, vaginal secretions, urine, stools or blood. Paediatric staff are probably more acquainted with congenital CMV infection but this is much rarer, affecting only 0.2–2% of live births in developed countries. In contrast, by the end of childhood, 50–80% of children will be seropositive for CMV infection. In many this will have been asymptomatic. In some young children, primary CMV infection may cause pneumonitis, hepatitis or a petechial rash and in older children and adolescents, CMV infection may cause a syndrome rather like glandular fever with fatigue, malaise, myalgia, headache, fever, hepatosplenomegaly, and jaundice with atypical lymphocytes on blood film. Recurrent infections are asymptomatic in the immunocompetent host.

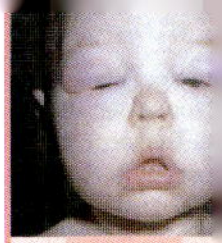

In contrast, in immunocompromised individuals, primary CMV disease is more likely to have clinical manifestations (including pneumonitis, hepatitis, chorioretinitis, gastrointestinal disease including mucosal ulceration, haemorrhage and perforation, pancreatitis, cholecystitis and neutropenia). Recurrent infection represents reactivation of latent infection (as with other members of the herpes virus family (i.e. herpes simplex, herpes varicella zoster and Epstein–Barr virus) or re-infection in someone who has previously had the disease.

Therefore, Ruth may be experiencing a primary CMV infection, or the CMV may have been transplanted by the donor organ, by blood transfusions or be reactivation by immunosuppression if she has had a previous infection.

How would you confirm the diagnosis?

CMV can be demonstrated in urine, saliva and tissues obtained by biopsy (e.g. renal biopsy of the transplanted kidney). Rapid detection is possible using monoclonal antibodies for CMV antigens or polymerase chain reaction for DNA. In an immunocompetent patient, primary infection is confirmed by the simultaneous detection of IgM as well as IgG antibodies. In immunocompromised patients, however, the distinction between primary and recurrent infections is more difficult as recurrent infections may be associated with excretion of CMV and even the presence of IgM antibodies. The demonstration of viraemia in blood culture, however, implies a worse prognosis regardless of whether the infection is primary or recurrent.

Can CMV infection be prevented in immunosuppressed patients?

In some transplantation regimes, CMV intravenous immunoglobulin is given within 72 hours of transplantation and once weekly until 4 months after transplantation. However, there is little consensus on this. Seronegative transplant recipients may also be given CMV vaccine and although the vaccine does not protect renal transplant recipients from CMV infection, it appears to reduce the virulence of primary infection.

11

THE MUSCULOSKELETAL SYSTEM

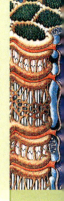

MUSCULOSKELETAL SYSTEM EXAMINATION SUMMARY

- **Do not forget to examine gait**
- **Is it sore anywhere?**
- **Look → Feel → Move → Measure**

INSPECTION

- As with the other systems observation is an essential part of the examination – thriving, splints, bandages, plaster casts, traction, wheelchair, limb deformities, etc.
- Always ask whether there is pain in the limbs or joints
- Start with the head and work down; begin with child sitting on edge of bed
- The degree of movement is measured from the neutral position

Neck

- Extension: 'Look up at the ceiling.'
- Flexion: 'Put your chin on your chest.'
- Lateral rotation: 'Look over your shoulder.'
- Lateral flexion: 'Put your ear on your shoulder.'

(**Never** ask a child to do a full rotation of their neck)

Temporomandibular joint

'Open your mouth as wide as possible and see if you can insert your second, third and fourth fingers into it.' If the joint is affected, crepitus can be felt

Shoulder joint

- Joint itself is too deep to see swelling or feel heat; need to stabilise the shoulder girdle
- All movements are tested passively
- Flexion, extension, abduction, superior and inferior rotation when abducted to 90°

Elbow joint

Look for swelling and feel for heat (comparing with other arm). Synovial swelling if present can be palpated below the lateral epicondyle as a boggy area; if not hot – chronic synovitis. Flexion and extension. Full extension = 180°; if unable to fully extend the patient has a fixed flexion deformity and is measured as the degrees short of 180°

Radioulnar joint

Pronation and supination with the elbow flexed and fixed to prevent shoulder movement

Wrist joint

- Inspect for swelling and heat over the dorsum
- Dorsiflexion (extension) and palmar flexion (flexion) = 90° each way
- Assess for stiffness at radial and ulnar joints

Metacarpophalangeal joints

- Palpate for swelling at the lateral surfaces of the joints
- Best way to assess movement: 'Make a fist' – should be able to bend fingers to 90° at all joints; also easier to observe for swelling between the joints when making a fist
- If distal interphalangeal joint swelling, look at the nails for pitting

Spine

With the child still sitting, so that the pelvis is splinted, ask the child to rotate the torso through 90° to assess rotation of the spine; flexion, extension, rotation and lateral flexion can be done at the end once the child is standing

Hip joint

Lie the child down. Like the shoulder joint the hip is too deep to assess for swelling or heat. Stabilise the pelvis then passively test abduction, adduction, flexion (holding down the opposite leg) and internal and external rotation (with the hip and knee at 90°)

Knee joint

This is the most frequently affected joint and the most commonly examined joints in exams:

- Look for the absence of indentations at the side of the patella indicating effusion
- Look for valgus and varus deformities
- Feel for heat and effusions (patellar tap)
- Extension: 'Push down on my hand.' Can squash hand if normal extension
- Flexion: 'Bend your knee and pull your heel up towards your bottom.'

(Ligament stability is not usually tested in the exam situation)

Ankle joint (3 joints)

- Look for swelling from behind, i.e. absence of indentations on either side of Achilles tendon
- Tibiotalar joint: dorsiflexion and plantar flexion
- Subtalar joint: inversion and eversion, stabilise the lower leg and rock the heel back and forward
- Midtarsal joints: medial and lateral movements of the foot

Metatarsal joints

Look for dactylitis

MEASURE

Limb circumference is measured from a set point above and below the tibial tuberosity to look for muscle wasting. Leg lengths are also important as arthritis of the knee will cause increased growth of that limb which will result in a scoliosis

- True leg length: anterior superior iliac spine to medial malleolus
- Apparent leg length: pubic symphysis to medial malleolus

SCOLIOSIS

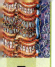

Inspect from behind with child standing. Describe the side of the scoliosis as the side to which the spine is convex. The shoulder on the convex side is elevated. Ask the child – 'Can you touch your toes?'

- If scoliosis disappears = *postural*, e.g. idiopathic (adolescent female), unilateral muscle spasm secondary to pain, unequal leg length
- If fixed = *structural*, e.g. idiopathic, Marfan's, neurofibromatosis, muscular dystrophy
- Associations:
  - — Sprengel's shoulder: high scapula ± cervical rib ± brachial nerve problems
  - — Klippel–Feil syndrome: fusion of cervical spine > short neck (differential diagnosis, Turner's syndrome)

LIMP

- Look for deformities, scars, rashes, joint swelling, etc.
- Ask the child to walk
- Are the leg lengths equal?
- Site of problem – need to examine hip, knee and ankle

MUSCULOSKELETAL SYSTEM SHORT CASES

PSORIATIC ARTHROPATHY

STEM: Rebecca is a 15-year-old girl who often complains of sore fingers. Please examine her.

PRESENTATION OF EXAMINATION FINDINGS

Rebecca is a 15-year-old girl with asymmetrical polyarthritis of the distal interphalangeal joints. She has no swelling of the large joints. On examination of her skin she has erythematous plaques with a thick silvery white scale, predominantly on her elbows, buttocks and scalp. She has mild pitting of her fingernails.

Thinking pause.....

Rebecca has psoriasis with psoriatic arthropathy.

How does psoriatic arthropathy differ from juvenile chronic arthritis?

The major difference between psoriatic arthropathy and JCA is the absence of systemic manifestations including fevers, generalised lymphadenopathy, hepatosplenomegaly or cardiac involvement.

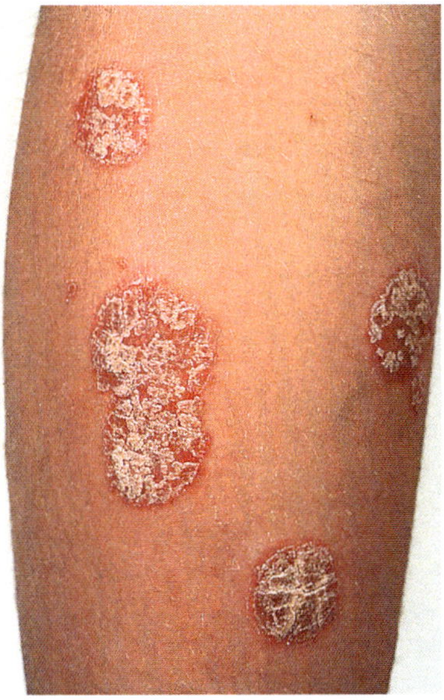

Fig. 11.1 *Typical plaque psoriasis.*
(Reproduced with kind permission from Schachner L A, Hansen R C. Pediatric Dermatology, 3rd edn. Edinburgh: Mosby, 2003.)

What tests could you do to help with the diagnosis of psoriatic arthropathy?

Patients with juvenile psoriatic arthritis are rheumatoid factor negative and there is an increased incidence of HLA B17 in psoriasis with peripheral arthritis; some patients have an increase of HLA B27 in the spondylitis group.

(For the management of psoriasis, more detail is provided in Case 3, Chapter 12.)

JUVENILE IDIOPATHIC ARTHRITIS

STEM: Nicholas is an 8-year-old boy who presented with a high fever and malaise 18 months ago. The fever was associated with a salmon-coloured rash. Examine his joints.

PRESENTATION OF EXAMINATION FINDINGS

Nicholas is an 8-year-old boy with symmetrical swelling of his wrists, knees and ankles. His metacarpophalangeal and proximal interphalangeal joints bilaterally are grossly swollen and deformed, with relative sparing of the distal interphalangeal joints. The joints are swollen, non-tender and not hot. Nicholas has limitation of movement of these joints, with particularly reduced function of his hands. He is afebrile and has no significant lymphadenopathy or hepatosplenomegaly. There is no rash present but he

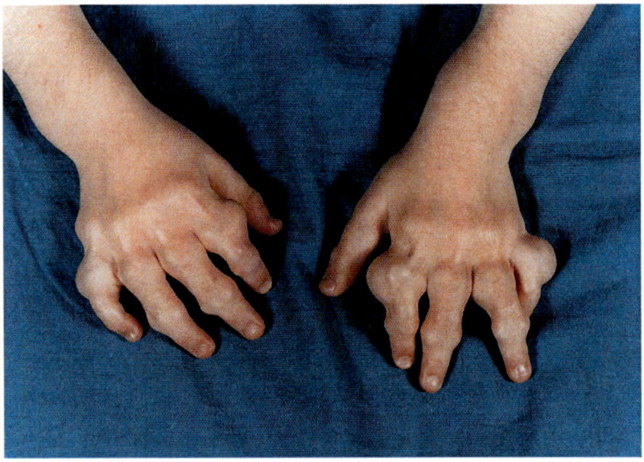

Fig. 11.2 *A boy with juvenile idiopathic arthritis showing marked deformity of the hands bilaterally. He has symmetrical swelling of the metacarpophalangeal joints. There is also bilateral swelling at the wrist joints.*

does have evidence of repeated subcutaneous injections in his upper thighs and arms. Nicholas has a port-a-cath in situ. I would like to plot his height and weight on a growth chart appropriate for his age and sex as he appears to be of short stature for an 8-year-old boy.

Thinking pause.....

Nicholas is an 8-year-old boy with systemic juvenile idiopathic polyarticular arthritis (JIA). It is likely that Nicholas requires frequent hospital admission and medication, possibly with methotrexate, in view of the port-a-cath.

Anything else?

I would like to assess his mobility and functional ability and to ask him how he manages at school.

How would you classify JIA?

JIA is by definition swelling of one or more joints for more than 6 months, in the absence of underlying pathology:

- Systemic
- Polyarticular: RF positive, RF negative
- Oligoarticular: persistent, extended
- Enthesitis related
- Others: psoriatic, IBD.

What investigations would you undertake?

In the acute phase, patients show elevated acute phase proteins, with raised ESR, CRP, SAA (serum amyloid A); platelets are also frequently raised. Patients are often anaemic. The presence of rheumatoid factor, other autoantibodies and HLA typing also help to classify the disease.

How would you manage this patient?

Management of JIA is with a multidisciplinary team involving physiotherapists and occupational therapists, chiropodists and orthotics together with physicians. Some patients may also require surgical input and support from psychologists and psychiatrists.

What is the mainstay of drug management?

This is a stepwise programme depending upon the severity and extent of the illness:

1. NSAIDS
2. Steroids:
   — oral prednisolone
   — IV methylprednisolone
   — intra-articular – triamcinolone hexacetamide
3. Immunosuppressants:
   — methotrexate
   — sulfasalazine – enthesitis
   — anti-TNF
   — sandoglobulin.

12
SKIN

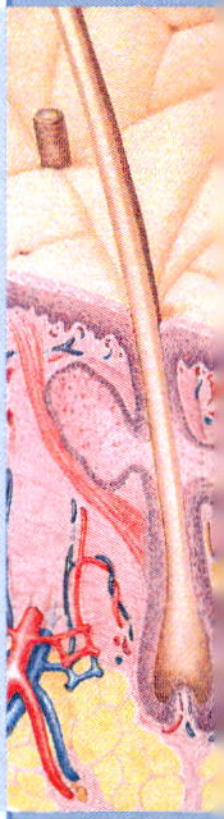

SHORT CASES FOR SKIN CONDITIONS

STEVENS–JOHNSON SYNDROME SECONDARY TO LAMOTRIGINE

STEM: Caroline is a 14-year-old girl with epilepsy who had been well controlled on sodium valproate. This medication had been weaned off as she had been seizure-free for 2 years. She subsequently had two further seizures. As she was a teenage girl, the increased risks of polycystic ovary syndrome and neural tube defects in pregnancy in women receiving sodium valproate were discussed with Caroline and her mother. In one study of 238 women, 27% of those who received sodium valproate over the age of 20 and 80% of those who received sodium valproate before the age of 20 demonstrated polycystic ovaries or increased serum testosterone. In many women the polycystic changes disappeared from the ovaries after the valproate therapy was stopped. There are also reports of amenorrhoea, irregular menstrual cycle and infertility. It was decided to re-commence her on anticonvulsants but to replace her previous sodium valproate with lamotrigine. A few days ago the dose of her lamotrigine was increased to 30 mg twice a day and she presented to the paediatric ward. Please examine her skin.

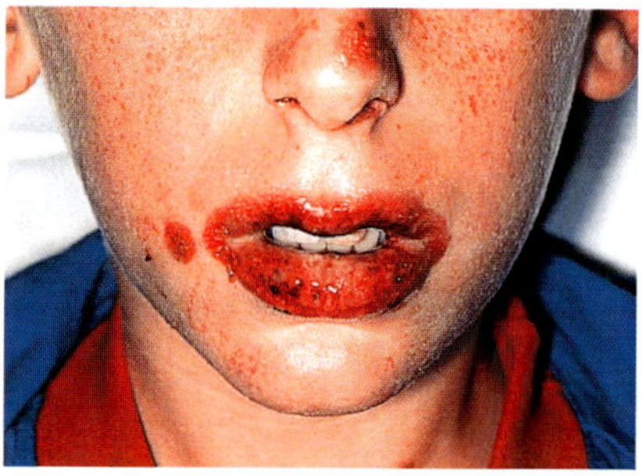

Fig. 12.1 *Stevens–Johnson syndrome showing severe ulceration of the mouth.* (Reproduced with kind permission from Lissauer T, Clayden G. Illustrated Textbook of Paediatrics, 2nd edn. Edinburgh: Mosby, 2001. Courtesy of Rob Primhak.)

PRESENTATION OF EXAMINATION FINDINGS

Caroline has developed extensive bullous lesions over her skin, purulent conjunctivitis, sore lips and a sore mouth and I can see from her observations chart that she has a pyrexia.

Thinking pause .....

This girl has developed unusual clinical features after recent exposure to a relatively new drug.

What is the most likely cause of her illness?

Antiepileptic drugs (AEDs) have the potential to cause many side effects. These side effects can be grouped into those which are dose dependent and common to most antiepileptic drugs:

- lethargy and drowsiness
- ataxia
- nausea and vomiting.

Each antiepileptic drug may also have side effects which are idiosyncratic to that drug. For example:

- phenytoin can cause gingival hypertrophy and hirsutism
- sodium valproate can cause hyperammonaemia, increased appetite and weight gain
- carbamazepine can cause blood dyscrasias.

Furthermore, many antiepileptic drugs have the capacity to interact with other anticonvulsants and other classes of drug, for example:

- Carbamazepine, phenobarbital and sodium valproate lower the concentration of most other anticonvulsant drugs.
- However, phenytoin may raise the plasma concentration of phenobarbital, and sodium valproate may raise the plasma concentration of ethosuximide.
- The effectiveness of oral contraceptives is reduced by interaction with drugs that induce hepatic enzyme activity (e.g. carbamazepine, phenytoin, phenobarbital, topiramate).

Finally, there is an increased risk of neural tube defect in pregnancy associated in particular with carbamazepine, phenytoin and sodium valproate. To counteract the risk of neural tube defects, folate supplements are advised for women before and during pregnancy. There is also an increased risk of neonatal bleeding associated with vitamin K deficiency in babies born to mothers receiving carbamazepine, phenobarbital and phenytoin during pregnancy.

What is the most likely diagnosis?

A diagnosis of Stevens–Johnson syndrome secondary to lamotrigine. Dose-dependent side effects of lamotrigine include a measles-like skin rash (particularly if used in conjunction with sodium valproate) and this usually arises within the first 3 weeks of commencing therapy. However, more rarely a full blown Stevens–Johnson syndrome may occur.

How would you manage this patient?

Stevens–Johnson syndrome can be very painful and there is also a significant risk of dehydration because of fluid loss through the skin lesions.

1. Lamotrigine was stopped.
2. Caroline was commenced on intravenous fluids.
3. Analgesia was given via a patient controlled analgesic system to deliver intravenous morphine.

4. She was also commenced on IV ranitidine because of slightly blood-stained vomit.
5. Dermatological treatment was with topical emollients.
6. Intravenous ceftriaxone was commenced to cover the very real possibility of secondary bacterial infection.

Mucosal involvement is a major problem in Stevens–Johnson syndrome but much less obvious than the external skin lesions. Mucosal involvement can be subtle but hidden mucosal involvement can manifest with vomiting, haematemesis and abdominal pain. Another feature of mucosal involvement may be distressing dysuria through urethral involvement. Topical lidocaine (lignocaine) gel may ease some of this urethral discomfort.

Subsequently Caroline was treated for her nausea and vomiting with intravenous ondansetron because the risk of extrapyramidal side effects in teenage girls are less with this drug than with metoclopramide.

Caroline was also reviewed by an ophthalmologist who found no evidence of corneal ulceration. She was commenced on steroid eye drops for her conjunctivitis.

Post script

Caroline made a full recovery and was subsequently re-started on sodium valproate.

HYPOPIGMENTED SKIN LESION

STEM: Charlie is an 8-year-old boy who has had a number of admissions for wheeze since the age of 2 years and had subsequently been diagnosed with asthma. At the age of 8 years, he was started on inhaled steroid prophylaxis for his asthma, following which pale areas on his chest were noticed. His mother attributed these to his steroid asthma therapy which she had discontinued. He was otherwise fit and well and there was no family history of autoimmune disease.

PRESENTATION OF EXAMINATION FINDINGS

Charlie has developed depigmented areas of skin, spreading over his chest, abdomen and neck.

Thinking pause.....
This is known as vitiligo.

What is the differential diagnosis of skin depigmentation in childhood?

Skin hypopigmentation may be localised or generalised and is obviously more apparent in dark-skinned children.

Local hypopigmentation includes:

- previous inflammation (e.g. chickenpox or eczema)
- burn or scar
- vitiligo.

Vitiligo is usually bilateral and symmetrical and may be associated with alopecia areata and other autoimmune diseases. Vitiligo is a circumscribed hypomelanosis resulting from enlarging and coalescing white macules, appears in a mirror-image distribution around body orifices, over the bony prominences (e.g. knees, elbows, hands), in the axillae and groins. It is familial in over one-third of cases and is often associated with a variety of autoimmune disorders.

Conditions associated with vitiligo include:

- Endocrine disorders: hyperthyroidism, hypothyroidism, diabetes mellitus, Addison's disease, hypoparathyroidism
- Skin diseases: morphoea, lichen sclerosus, alopecia areata, malignant melanoma
- Other conditions: pernicious anaemia, myasthenia gravis
- Tuberous sclerosis (the lesions are typically ash-leaf in shape. Other skin stigmata include a shagreen patch, a thickened area of skin over the lumbosacral area, small fibromata under the toenails, adenoma sebaceum on the face beyond the age of 5 and occasionally darker brown café-au-lait patches anywhere on the skin)
- Pityriasis versicolor (a fungal infection)
- Pityriasis alba (usually the cheeks and sometimes upper arms and accompanied by scaling).

Generalised hypopigmentation includes:

- albinism (pink pupils, blue irises and white hair)
- phenylketonuria (blond hair and blue eyes)
- hypopituitarism (short stature and micropenis).

Could the hypopigmentation be related to inhaled steroids?

Hypopigmentation is not a recognised side effect of inhaled or systemic steroids. Inhaled steroids are preferred to oral steroids because the systemic dose is smaller and, therefore, systemic side effects are less common. Oral candidiasis can occur following the use of inhaled steroids and high-dose inhaled steroids can lead to suppression of the endogenous hypopituitary adrenal axis and stunting of growth (see Case 1, Ch. 9).

What investigations would you undertake?

The full blood count showed an ESR of 3 mm/hour (normal), with normal haemoglobin, white cell count and platelet count. Autoantibody screen showed a weakly positive antinuclear antibody. This is unusual in this age group and may occur with autoimmune connective tissue disease and also with certain infections. However, ENA (extractable nuclear antigen) antibody screen for RNP, Sm, La and Ro were all negative. The normal ESR is very much against systemic autoimmune disease.

Double-stranded DNA antibody level was 4 international units/ml (negative).

Post script

Clinically Charlie was thought to have vitiligo and was referred to the Dermatology Department who noted that he had had eczema in the past but agreed that the lesions looked typical of vitiligo apart from the fact that the loss of pigment was not complete in the affected areas.

PSORIASIS

> **STEM:** Graham is a 14-year-old boy who has presented to his GP with the appearance of a rash. On further questioning, he admits to having had a sore throat in the previous fortnight. Please examine him.

PRESENTATION OF EXAMINATION FINDINGS

Graham has striated lesions over his left shoulder and left arm, each covered with a thick, silvery white scale. There is also a single large lesion over the left elbow.

What is the most likely diagnosis?

Graham has psoriasis. Most commonly in childhood, psoriasis presents as an eruption of small (1 cm) slightly scaly, red lesions in a shower over the trunk. This often follows a streptococcal sore throat and most presentations are in older childhood. This so-called guttate psoriasis usually clears spontaneously in around 6–10 weeks but in a smaller number of children, psoriasis persists. Psoriatic lesions are not itchy and the differential diagnosis of scaly skin lesions is shown in Table 12.1. Guttate psoriasis is most often confused with pityriasis rosea. However, the oval patches of pityriasis rosea are larger and there may be a characteristic herald patch.

About one-third of all childhood presentations of psoriasis are the guttate form but in two-thirds of cases, the pattern is more like that in adults. Instead of there being a large shower of lesions all over the trunk, the condition is largely confined to the knees, elbows, scalp, eyebrows and extensor surfaces.

Why are Graham's lesions in a striated pattern?

Psoriasis is one of the conditions which demonstrates the Koebner phenomena in which trauma to previously unaffected skin results in fresh lesions. Although psoriasis is not itself itchy, Graham presumably scratched his arm for some other reason and the psoriasis then appeared at these sites. Examples of the Koebner phenomena are:

- psoriasis
- lichen planus
- the rash of systemic onset juvenile chronic arthritis.

Table 12.1 Causes of a scaly skin

Condition	Clinical feature	Inheritance
Collodion baby	Rare, severe, present at birth	Sporadic
Ichthyosis vulgaris	Commonly widespread, spares flexures	Autosomal dominant
Sex-linked ichthyosis	Coarser with brown scales and not sparing flexures	Sex-linked
Keratosis pilaris	Around hair follicles, upper thighs, arms and buttocks, onset puberty	Sporadic
Darier's disease	Rare, follicular, greasy scales, neck and upper trunk	Autosomal dominant
Psoriasis	Guttate or extensor	Family history +
Pityriasis rosea	Herald spot, body rash, ? infection	Sporadic

Koebner phenomena may not be so obvious, the rash arising where the skin has been rubbed (e.g. from the pressure of underclothing).

How would you manage this patient?

Treatment may be difficult in children as many of the more potent adult therapies cannot be used safely. Topical corticosteroid or coal tar preparations are commonly used but these may smell strongly and discolour clothing. Thickened psoriasis on the scalp can be treated with coal tar shampoo. Dithranol can be used for large plaques on extensor surfaces but oral retinoids, psoralens, ultraviolet light and cytotoxics should be avoided in childhood. In some cases, however, graduated UVB light exposure may be used under the supervision of a dermatologist.

What are the complications of psoriasis?

Teenagers can also develop psoriatic arthropathy but this is extremely uncommon. Nail involvement is usually confined to minor pitting of the nail. Specific nails may be involved rather than all the finger- and toenails. Generalised pustular psoriasis is rare in childhood but such children may need admission to hospital for monitoring of fluid and electrolyte balance and treatment of secondary infection. Such widespread lesions can lead to large amounts of fluid loss via the skin.

What advice would you give to the parents?

There is a genetic element to psoriasis and, in some patients, recurrences of psoriasis seem to be provoked by episodes of stress. The parents and child should be aware of this from the outset and paediatricians need to be aware of the social stigma that can arise. Graham was particularly anxious as he had already suffered some name calling at school when changing for rugby.

ECZEMA

STEM: Angus is a 1-year-old boy who is brought to see you in clinic by his mother. She already sees you because her older child has asthma. Angus has had dry skin since birth but this has become worse recently and itching has led to bleeding. Please examine him.

PRESENTATION OF EXAMINATION FINDINGS

On examination Angus has the typical erythematous itchy, weeping rash of eczema. There are also skin cracks behind the pinnae of both ears and scratching has led to some excoriation. He has lesions on both cheeks, over his chest and on the extensor surfaces of his forearms and knees.

Thinking pause.....
This is the typical presentation of an infant with eczema.

What advice would you give to the parents?
You should first tell the parents that you have made a diagnosis of eczema which is the commonest itchy skin disease in childhood affecting up to 10% of primary school age children. There is an association with asthma, hay fever and food intolerance in three-quarters of families and you may wish to enquire about this further. Three-quarters of cases begin before the age of around 2 years and although many children will grow out of their eczema to some extent by school age or in adolescence, they will always be prone to contact dermatitis and may continue to have generally dry skin (atopic xerosis). Early onset and severe disease in childhood make the prognosis less good. You should give advice on home management as summarised in Box 12.1.

Could there be any other cause?
Some doctors are confused because, as in Angus' case, the initial presentation is predominantly on the extensor surfaces. However, the distribution of atopic eczema varies with the age of the child. Extensor eczema is more typical in early life but beyond the age of 2 years atopic eczema then has a predilection for the skin flexures, especially behind the knees, the front of elbows and around the neck. Other causes of itching lesions are listed in Box 12.2 but these are unlikely to be confused with atopic eczema.

Is there anything else you should tell the family?
Ectopic eczema is a chronic relapsing condition for which there is no cure. It may help the family to know that there are genetic factors over which they have no control. Many more children have dry skin and eczema in infancy than in older childhood and this may be reassuring. A child with eczema should avoid contact (particularly kissing) with someone who has a cold

Box 12.1 Home management of the child with eczema

1. The family should use only non-biological washing powder.
2. The child's nails should be kept cut short.
3. It may be necessary for the child to wear cotton mittens at night to prevent scratching.
4. Do not use perfumed soaps or bubble baths.
5. The child should wear only cotton garments next to the skin.
6. Emollients (moisturisers) such as E45 aqueous cream can be applied liberally to all body areas and have no side effects whatsoever.
7. Baby oil can be added to a daily cool bath provided it is not perfumed.
8. 1% hydrocortisone ointment can be used on all but the very smallest infants even on the face. Ointment is better for chronic dry eczema, cream for moist eczema. More potent steroids (Eumovate, Betnovate and Dermovate in ascending order of strength) may require dermatological advice and the prescriber should be aware that growth suppression is possible if there are large areas of skin involvement. Furthermore, in older children, who may have associated asthma or hay fever, the total daily steroid dose will be the accumulation of that absorbed through the skin, that absorbed through the lungs from metered dose inhalers, any absorbed through the nasal mucosa from nasal sprays to treat rhinitis and any oral steroids used for acute exacerbation of asthma.
9. If there is secondary infection, topical treatment with oxytetracycline or fusidic acid ointment (Fucidin) may be necessary.
10. There is little evidence to support dietary restriction. If the parents think that particular items in the diet exacerbate eczema, then an 8-week trial of elimination of that specific food may be justified. The most likely foodstuffs are egg and dairy milk products.

Box 12.2 Causes of itching

- Eczema
- Contact dermatitis
- Some drug reactions
- Conjugated hyperbilirubinaemia
- Kidney failure
- Scabies
- Papular urticaria
- Animal mites
- Flea bites
- Lice infestations (pediculosis)

sore as there is the risk of developing widespread eczema herpeticum from herpes simplex infection. The parents should be told that if the eczema suddenly deteriorates for no apparent reason, the child should be seen promptly as this may be the first sign of secondary infection. If secondary infection does not respond to topical antibiotics, then oral flucloxacillin (or erythromycin if penicillin allergic) may be necessary.

HYPERPIGMENTED SKIN

STEM: You are asked to see Wilson, a newborn term infant, on the postnatal wards because the parents are distraught because he has a birth mark on his face. His father is Afro-Caribbean and his mother is Caucasian. Wilson is their first child. Please examine him.

PRESENTATION OF EXAMINATION FINDINGS

Wilson has a giant melanocytic naevus over most of his forehead and on examination there are no other abnormalities.

Thinking pause.....

It is difficult to reassure the parents because the lesion is so striking and will not be hidden by clothing or hair. You must be honest with them that there is no easy treatment or cure for this. In addition, there is a small risk of malignant transformation. Malignant melanoma is fortunately extremely rare in childhood but when it does occur it is often in conjunction with a congenital giant melanocytic naevus, more typically in the bathing trunk region.

What are the causes of increased pigmentation?

These are listed in Table 12.2. Few occur in the newborn period.

The most common cause in childhood is postinflammation. In postpubertal individuals with proven neurofibromatosis type I, 75% have 6 or more café-au-lait spots of more than 1.5 cm diameter. Among normal people, 10% have 1–5 café-au-lait spots of more than 1.5 cm size. In normal children under 5 years of age, only 0.75% have more than 2 café-au-lait macules larger than 1.5 cm.

What further action would you take in Wilson's case?

Wilson should have an MRI scan to exclude intracranial extension of this pigmented lesion.

Post script

The MRI was normal. Wilson was referred to a dermatologist and a plastic surgeon. Both agreed that there was no further treatment and that although plastic surgery was something that Wilson might want to consider himself when old enough to give consent, this was not appropriate at present.

Table 12.2 Causes of pigmentation

Type	Description	Onset
Racial	Generalised	Birth
UVL exposure	Light exposed	Any age
Freckles	1–4 mm pale brown macules on light-exposed areas	2 years onset
Lentigines	1–4 mm dark macules; generalised; often after light exposure	Later childhood
Leopard syndrome	Lentigines, ECG abnormalities, ocular defects, pulmonary stenosis, abnormal genitalia, retarded growth, deafness	Birth onwards
Café-au-lait spots	1–4 cm oval macules, less than six in total	2 years onwards
Neurofibromatosis	Numerous café-au-lait spots; steady increase in number; axillary accentuation	2 years onwards
Postinflammatory	At site of injury or other skin disease	Later childhood
Acanthosis nigricans	Pale pigmentation and velvety thickening in flexures; autosomal dominant; can also occur with hyperinsulinism	2 years onwards
Urticaria pigmentosa	Pale brown 0.5–1 cm macules which urticate on scratching; increase in number	Birth onwards
Albright's syndrome	Polyostotic fibrous dysplasia and sexual precocity in females	Childhood
Peutz–Jeghers syndrome	Pigmented spots in or around the mouth often associated with gastrointestinal bleeding	Childhood onwards
Haemosiderosis	e.g. Multiple transfusions for thalassaemia	Usually teenager onwards
Addison's disease	When the pigmentation may be confined to the palmar creases or to the buccal mucosa	Any age
Primary biliary cirrhosis	Older child, usually a girl	Later childhood

INCONTINENTIA PIGMENTOSA

STEM: Sally is a term newborn baby girl who you are asked to see on the postnatal ward because the midwife has noticed blisters on her arm. Please examine her.

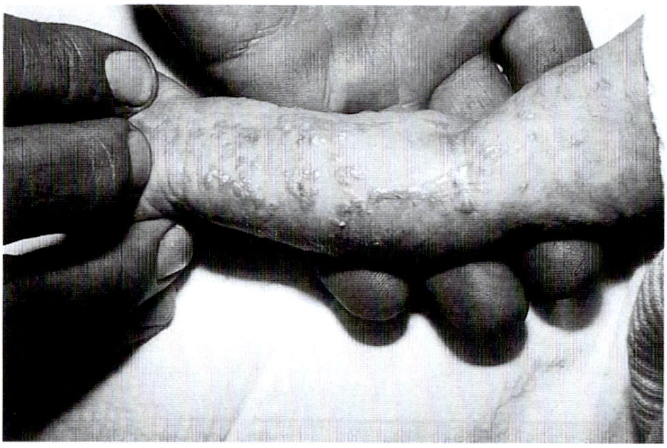

Fig. 12.2 *Incontinentia pigmentosa: vesicular stage.*
(Reproduced with kind permission from McIntosh N, Helms P J, Smyth R L (eds) Forfar & Arneil's Textbook of Pediatrics, 6th edn. Edinburgh: Churchill Livingstone, 2003. Courtesy of Maureen Rogers.)

PRESENTATION OF EXAMINATION FINDINGS

Sally is a baby with linear groups of vesicular lesions on her left arm. She is otherwise well and does not appear to be septic. I would like to ask her parents whether she has any history of herpes simplex infection, particularly genital herpes.

Thinking pause.....
In view of the linear nature of the vesicles in an otherwise well baby my impression would be that this baby may have incontinentia pigmentosa.

What other diagnoses would you consider?

There are many causes of blistering lesions in childhood (Box 12.3) but very few of these are present at birth. The only other common blistering conditions in the newborn are the various types of epidermolysis bullosa, neonatal herpes simplex, and neonatal impetigo which is usually a staphylococcal infection.

What can you tell me about incontinentia pigmentosa?

Classically, there are four cutaneous stages of incontinentia pigmentosa. The vesicular lesions at birth (stage I) disappear spontaneously over several weeks. However, stage II is the appearance of linear, warty lesions which

Box 12.3 Common vesicular/pustular rashes in childhood

Cause	Features
Varicella/zoster virus	Simple chickenpox is characterised by polymorphic lesions, i.e. papules, vesicles and pustules, which usually present at the same stage. Shingles usually has a dermatomal pattern, or it may be widespread in the immunocompromised
Herpes simplex	Neonatal herpes simplex may present as blisters and pustules in the newborn and requires urgent treatment with aciclovir. Primary herpes simplex usually presents as mouth ulceration and systemic upset. Secondary herpes simplex presents as clusters of vesicles
Hand/foot/mouth disease	Vesicles or grey pustules on palms, soles and back of mouth (Coxsackie A 16)
Scabies	Vesicles/pustules usually on feet and axillary region in young babies. Finger webs in the older child. Excoriations +++ and secondary infection common. Others usually affected
Eczema	Eczema has many causes but acute eczema is characterised by vesicles especially on the sides of the fingers and palms of the hand
Impetigo	Clusters of 1–2 cm flaccid blisters quickly rupture and dry with honey-coloured crusts
Epidermolysis bullosa	Autosomal recessive forms are severe whereas autosomal dominant forms are milder. Look for old scars and nail deformities
Incontinentia pigmentosa	Affects only girls. Look for old scars, hyperpigmented whorls and dental abnormalities
Dermatitis herpetiformis	Usually confined to buttocks or genitalia
Erythema multiforme	Rarely

arise between 1 and 4 months of age and may occur on the limbs or on the trunk. In stage III these warty lesions are replaced by whorls or brown pigmentation following Blaschko's lines on the trunk. This is macular hyperpigmentation and usually appears between the first and second year of life. These lesions persist until early adult life. Stage IV comprises linear hypopigmented streaks with alopecia, particularly on the lower legs.

Other dermatological features of incontinentia pigmentosa are alopecia and nail dystrophy. Non-dermatological features include epilepsy, learning difficulties, cerebral palsy (neurological abnormalities in about 30%), strabismus, cataracts, retinal detachment (ocular abnormalities in 30%) and

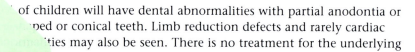

... of children will have dental abnormalities with partial anodontia or peg-shaped or conical teeth. Limb reduction defects and rarely cardiac abnormalities may also be seen. There is no treatment for the underlying condition.

Inheritance is believed to be X-linked dominant and the condition is only seen in girls as it is thought to be lethal in males in utero.

GUM HYPERTROPHY

STEM: Gabriella is a 14-year-old girl who has moved to your area from another part of the country. She was first diagnosed with generalised epilepsy at the age of 2 and has been on a number of anticonvulsants but for the last decade has been on phenytoin. Her current dose is 300 mg orally twice a day. She has become self-conscious about some of the side effects which are developing from the medication and her parents enquire whether her anticonvulsant should be changed. Please examine her.

PRESENTATION OF EXAMINATION FINDINGS

Gabriella has gum hypertrophy, with no evidence of mucosal bleeding or infective gingivitis. She also has facial hirsutism. She is otherwise well with no evidence of any other drug-related side effects.

Thinking pause.....

This girl has developed two of the recognised chronic adverse effects associated with phenytoin therapy. In addition to the usual dose-dependent adverse effects common to most anticonvulsant drugs (nystagmus, ataxia, lethargy) each of the antiepileptic drugs has its own particular side effects. Chronic use of phenytoin is associated with gum hypertrophy, hirsutism, coarse facies, osteomalacia and megaloblastic anaemia due to folate deficiency.

Should you consider any other causes of gum hypertrophy?

Given the hirsutism, a phenytoin side effect is the most likely cause. Nevertheless, periodontal disease is common in the population and should be considered. Periodontal disease leads to gingivitis with red and swollen gums which bleed easily. Bad oral hygiene may lead to dental plaques and food residue trapped between the teeth, both of which may give rise to inflammation of the gums. In contrast, swelling of the gums is less common than periodontal disease and is associated with a number of problems in addition to the commonly recognised association with phenytoin therapy, for example:

- puberty
- pregnancy
- other drugs such as nifedipine

- amyloidosis
- acute myeloid leukaemia
- scurvy
- Vincent's disease (acute ulcerative gingivitis).

An important distinguishing factor between periodontal disease leading to gingivitis and simple gum hypertrophy is that in the latter the gums are not inflamed and do not bleed on contact. Scurvy can lead to a combination of both gingivitis and gum hypertrophy. Vincent's disease is classically caused by combined infection with *Borrelia vincentii* and *Fusobacterium nucleatum*. It is seen in adolescence rather than childhood and risk factors include poor nutrition and smoking. It may be associated with halitosis.

PETECHIAE

STEM: Katie is a toddler of 18 months who was rushed to the Accident and Emergency Department by ambulance yesterday evening because her parents noticed pinhead-sized blood spots under her skin which did not blanch when they pressed a glass upon them (the tumbler test). The history is that Katie has had a troublesome cough for the last week with an intermittent fever but no other symptoms. Her 4-year-old brother has also had similar symptoms. Katie is fully immunised including the pertussis immunisation. Please examine her.

PRESENTATION OF EXAMINATION FINDINGS

On examination she seems well with a temperature of 37.7°C, mild tachypnoea of 36 breaths per minute, some intercostal recession and a mixture of crepitations and expiratory wheeze. The only other examination finding is that there are multiple petechiae over her upper chest, under her chin and on both cheeks.

Thinking pause.....

Katie has a petechial rash on her upper trunk associated with a mild lower respiratory tract infection but is otherwise relatively well.

What is the most likely diagnosis?

In the UK, young children presenting with a combination of crepitations and wheeze in mid winter are most likely to have bronchiolitis, the commonest cause of which is respiratory syncytial virus. The petechiae are confined to the distribution of the superior vena cava and are most likely cough petechiae due to raised intrathoracic pressure. The parents were rightly concerned that a rash which does not blanch with the tumbler test could be a sign of meningococcal septicaemia and any GP seeing such a rash is recommended to give parenteral benzylpenicillin before transfer to hospital. If the petechiae are not confined to the distribution of the superior vena cava then abnormal bleeding must be considered (Table 12.3).

Table 12.3 Causes of abnormal bleeding

Abnormality	Outcome	Features
Platelets	Thrombocytopenia	*Decreased production:* generalised bone marrow failure, including leukaemia; specific megakaryocyte failure, usually following viral infection (including congenital) but also inherited forms or associated with syndromes *Increased destruction:* immunological (ITP or ATP); DIC (including HUS); Kasabach–Merritt syndrome (giant haemangioma); hypersplenism; Wiskott–Aldrich syndrome (eczema and prone to infection)
	Normal platelet count but abnormal platelet function	Von Willebrand's disease
Clotting factors	Decreased or abnormal production	Vitamin K deficiency Malabsorption, liver disease and warfarin all deplete factors II, VII, IX, X Haemophilia A and Von Willebrand's disease (factor VIII) Haemophilia B (factor IX), i.e. Christmas disease
	Antagonism Consumption	Heparin DIC (including HUS)
Vascular endothelium	HSP Infections, especially meningococcaemia (perhaps DIC also)	

How would you manage a child with presumed meningococcal infection?

The febrile child with generalised petechiae or purpura should be presumed to have meningococcal infection until proven otherwise. The most urgent needs are to treat shock and to start a broad-spectrum antibiotic while awaiting cultures and sensitivities before changing to intravenous penicillin. Meningococcal disease can present with meningitis or sepsis or both. The rash may appear at any time in the illness and may be petechial, purpuric, ecchymotic or necrotic. The rash may be macular or maculopapular and may appear anywhere on the body – face, palate, conjunctiva, trunk, pressure sites or the palms and soles. In up to one-third of cases, the rash is initially a maculopapular pink rash and not the typical petechial or purpuric rash. The petechial areas may coalesce and produce areas of

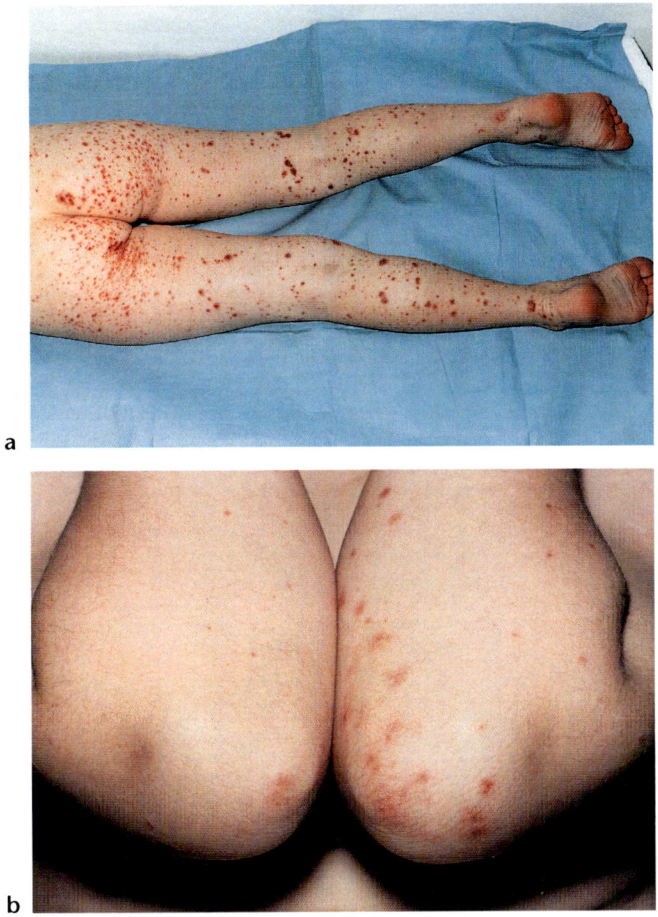

Fig. 12.3 *Petechial rash in Henoch–Schönlein purpura occurring on* (**a**) *the buttocks and extensor surfaces of the legs, and* (**b**) *the arms.*

necrosis especially at the peripheries such as fingers, toes and tips of the nose.

Henoch–Schönlein purpura (HSP) can appear almost as dramatic but the rash is usually confined to the buttocks and lower limbs (see Fig. 12.3) and though arthralgia can occur in both meningococcal disease and HSP, children with HSP are usually relatively well and certainly do not have hypotension or altered conscious level. Leukaemia can present as spontaneous bruising in the skin but there is usually associated pallor and often a longer history rather than an acute presentation. Accidental trauma very rarely gives rise to petechiae. Petechial bruising which is allegedly due to an accident should be treated with suspicion. The commonest cause of petechiae due to trauma is as the result of a slap mark and the petechiae may occur in linear patterns due to the imprint of a slap. Petechiae to the pinna of the ear are usually a result of a slap to the side of the head.

With which haematological disorders are petechiae most commonly associated?

Spontaneous petechiae are more commonly associated with platelet abnormalities. Abnormalities of platelets can also give rise to purpura, epistaxis, gastrointestinal bleeding or haematuria and retinal and intracranial haemorrhage. In contrast, abnormality of clotting factors classically gives rise to larger skin bruises following trivial trauma or bleeding into muscles or joints (haemarthrosis). However, abnormalities of clotting factors can also give rise to gastrointestinal and intracerebral bleeding (as in haemorrhagic disease of the newborn due to vitamin K deficiency). In vasculitis the purpura is palpable whereas in abnormalities of platelets and clotting factors, the lesions are usually macular.

Post script

Katie's platelet count was normal and although this does not exclude a coagulopathy due to abnormalities of clotting factors, no further investigations were undertaken as the petechiae were confined to the region of the superior vena cava.

INDEX

C

G

H

I

J

K

O

P

R

S